It's Not All in Your Head

It's Not All in Your Head

How Worrying about Your Health Could Be Making You Sick— and What You Can Do about It

Gordon J. G. Asmundson, PhD
Steven Taylor, PhD

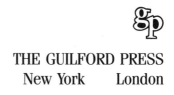

THE GUILFORD PRESS
New York   London

© 2005 The Guilford Press
A Division of Guilford Publications, Inc.
72 Spring Street, New York, NY 10012
www.guilford.com

The information in this volume is not intended as a substitute for consultation with health care professionals. Each individual's health concerns should be evaluated by a qualified professional.

Printed in the United States of America

This book is printed on acid-free paper.

Last digit is print number: 9   8   7   6   5   4   3

Library of Congress Cataloging-in-Publication Data

Asmundson, Gordon J. G.
     It's not all in your head: how worrying about your health could be making you sick—and what you can do about it / Gordon J. G. Asmundson, Steven Taylor.
          p.   cm.
     Includes bibliographical references and index.
     ISBN 1-57230-993-8 (pbk.) — ISBN 1-59385-146-4 (cloth)
     1. Health—Psychological aspects.   2. Compulsive behavior.   3. Health—Miscellanea.   I. Taylor, Steven, 1960–   II. Title.
     RC533.A85 2005
     616.85′84—dc22
                                                                          2004025955

To my amazing parents,
Calvin (who passed away during the writing of this book)
and Eileen, who taught me to soar,
and to my beautiful daughter and wife,
Aleiia and Kimberley,
who keep me well grounded
—G. J. G. A.

To Amy Sue Janeck and Alex Janeck Taylor
—S. T.

Contents

Part III

MAINTAINING YOUR GAINS

Acknowledgments

We would like to thank several people for their support during the writing of this book. Kitty Moore, Executive Editor, encouraged us to take on this project and made working with The Guilford Press a pleasure. The thoughtful critiques of Christine Benton and Ron and Judy Norton helped us improve the content and readability of many chapters. Thanks also to John Walker for generously sharing his time and ideas about the treatment of health anxiety and to the many patients who have taught us so much from their personal experiences with health anxiety. Last, but certainly not least, we are grateful to our families for their unwavering love and never-ending support during this project: Kimberley and Aleiia Asmundson, Amy Sue Janeck, and Alex Janeck Taylor (who was not yet born but was kicking like a soccer star at the time of writing).

Preface

Do you have symptoms that your doctor can't explain? Do you worry that there might be something seriously wrong with your body or about catching a disease? Or perhaps you know someone like this. If so, you're not alone. One of our patients, John, suffered each day from stinging pains in his chest. He thought there was something seriously wrong with his heart, and he worried about dying. To his surprise and dismay, his doctor could find no medical cause. John sought a second opinion and then a third and a fourth. Each time he was told there was nothing wrong. One doctor even had the nerve to tell John that his problems were "all in his head." Yet his pains persisted and, as a result, he stopped doing things that caused his heart to race and spent hours surfing the Internet for a possible explanation for the way he was feeling. His life started falling apart. Another patient, Debye, worried that she had stomach cancer. Debye feared that she would have a slow, painful death just like her mother, who had bravely struggled with cancer for years; Debye's painful cramps were real. She wasn't imagining them. But her doctors, including a cancer specialist, were unable to find a cause. John and Debye both had family and friends who were concerned but frustrated because they couldn't really understand what the root of the problem was or how to help.

We all have times when we worry about being sick or catching something that will make us sick. But some worry more than others. The critical questions are Do you worry too much about your health? and Do others tell you that you should stop worrying so much over nothing? About one in every five people worries a lot about his or her health, and this worry can sometimes be all consuming. It may be hard to tell when we're worrying too much, especially when we learn from an early age that changes in the way our bodies feel are things to be wary of, monitored, and checked by a doctor if persistent. Reading this book can help you decide whether anxiety is playing a role in your symptoms. If somebody you know worries a lot about his or her health, this book will aid you in understanding what the person is going through and will give you ideas for how you can help.

Debye's cramps were not caused by cancer. She was suffering from stomach upset from drinking too much coffee combined with the effects of being very anxious. *Misinterpretation* of her symptoms was, in fact, an important source of her problem. Thinking her cramps were a sign of cancer made Debye feel a great deal of anxiety and caused her many a sleepless night. People like John and Debye aren't suffering from a medical disease—they're suffering from what we call *health anxiety*. They worry a lot about physical symptoms that are part of the stresses of everyday life and *not* disease.

Even if you worry too much about your health, this *doesn't* mean the problem is "all in your head." Your symptoms are very real; it's just that they are not caused by a medical problem. Understandably, people usually resist this possibility at first. The good news is that you don't have anything to lose by considering whether anxiety could be contributing to what you're going through. If, after reading this book, you decide that you don't have an anxiety problem, you've learned something important. On the other hand, if you realize that you're suffering from too much worry about your physical symptoms, you've also learned something valuable. You'll have learned about what's causing your symptoms.

The really good news is that help is available, whether you worry a lot about your health or whether you're concerned about someone who does. There are proven, effective strategies for dealing with the experience of health anxiety. Sometimes the hardest step is the first one: understanding and coming to grips with what's wrong. Once you're over that hurdle you can learn and practice a number of strategies that will allow you to control your health anxiety and get on with living life. This book will help both you and your loved ones gain a better understanding of your health worries and ways to overcome them.

Part I

UNDERSTANDING HEALTH ANXIETY

One

Do I Worry Too Much about My Health?

way more days than not. Sometimes I also get headaches and feel clumsy. I've seen my family doctor as well as several specialists to try to find out what's wrong with me. At first I thought I might have the flu, but after feeling lousy for three weeks I began to worry that I might have Lou Gehrig's disease. My uncle died from it a few years ago. The neurologist gave me a whole bunch of tests, including an MRI, and assures me that I don't have Lou Gehrig's disease or multiple sclerosis. An internal medicine specialist thought it might be Hodgkin's disease, especially after I told her about my night sweats, but her tests also failed to find anything wrong. Now my family doctor assures me I probably have nothing to worry about. But something's not right with me. I'm not imagining my sluggishness, headaches, clumsiness, or night sweats. I've been reading a lot on the Internet about these symptoms. I think the doctors must have missed something. Maybe it *is* multiple sclerosis or even a brain tumor!"

Bob: "Dangerous germs are everywhere."

"For as long as I can remember, I've had a healthy habit of staying away from germs. They're everywhere—doorknobs, handrails, telephone receivers, ATM buttons, toilet seats, money—and really must be avoided. Other people have touched these things, and who knows where their hands have been or what diseases they have. I frequently see people who, with good intentions of stopping their germs from spreading, cup their hand over their face when coughing or sneezing. Good for them? No way! These same people take their unwashed, germ-infested hands and use them to operate the photocopier, twist open the lid to add some cream to their java, and greet coworkers with a friendly and germ-laden pat on the back. And that's just the start. What do you think happens when nature calls? The cough germs get spread to the bathroom door, the toilet seat, the flusher, and join the splash and spatter germs of those who've already completed their lavatory business. Most of my coworkers don't wash after flushing, and as a result their hands become a veritable germ party. Bathrooms are the worst for me. I try not to use them in public but, when this can't be avoided, I do most things with my feet—opening the doors, lifting or lowering the toilet seat, and operating the flusher. In the past few weeks I've started carrying latex gloves for those situations where I can't handle things with my foot technique. The gloves have proven useful in other situations, and I have started wearing them regularly. My family and friends tell me I'm too worried about germs and I have a germ phobia. I agree that I might be a little obsessed, but I think it's a healthy obsession."

We all worry about our health from time to time, often because we try to understand the reasons for the sensations our bodies are producing. Could my upset stomach be the result of something I ate, or is it an ulcer? Are my head-aches and sore eyes the result of a rough day, or do I have a brain tumor? What is that pain in my chest area? Could it be something wrong with my heart? Why have I been feeling so tired lately? Am I working too much, or could it be early signs of multiple sclerosis? We may worry about catching some sort of disease. For example, during the first few months of the severe acute respiratory syn-drome (SARS) outbreak in 2003, many people worried about being exposed to the virus after having encountered somebody with a cough. People who have or have had a serious disease, such as cancer or a heart condition, also may worry a great deal about their health. But some people worry too much. Joan, for exam-ple, worried about having colon cancer, even though she had seen three doctors who all told her she didn't. Joan's worries were excessive. It is estimated that about 20 percent of the population—one in every five people—worry too much about being sick.

If you're reading this book, it is a safe bet that your doctor or doctors have been unable to provide a satisfactory explanation for some of the bodily sensa-tions and disease-related questions that are causing you concern, let alone offer you any effective relief. Do you spend some time each day worrying about the causes of your bodily sensations? Are you afraid some sort of malfunction or physical breakdown is happening in your body and that you have an undiag-nosed disease? Do friends and family tell you that you worry too much about your health or call you a hypochondriac or germ phobic? Have your doctors told you there is nothing wrong and that you shouldn't worry? Maybe you aren't quite sure and you wonder, "Do I worry too much, or do I really have a serious dis-ease?" If so, this chapter will help you decide.

In the pages that follow, we suggest an alternative way of understanding the sensations that cause you concern. This is a necessary first step in helping you determine whether you worry too much about your health. We also ask you sev-eral questions and have you complete a self-assessment regarding your health-related worries. You will probably be skeptical at first of the alternative explana-tions we suggest. We know this from our experience with the many people we've seen in our research and clinical practice. The *cognitive-behavioral approach* we use asks you to consider that the bodily sensations that concern you might not be symptoms of disease but rather result from such things as stress and fatigue. Even if considered with the greatest of reluctance at first, our approach can be very effective in helping you identify your health-related worry and, where excessive, improve the many areas of your life that it affects. If other things haven't helped, isn't it worth a try?

What Is Health Anxiety?

Most cognitive-behavioral researchers and practitioners use the term *health anxi-ety* to describe the wide range of worry that people can have about their health.

Many of the questions you will be asked about have a specific focus on health anxiety. Thus, to help you fully understand how to determine whether you worry too much about your health, we first discuss the terms *health* and *anxiety*, as well as their combined use.

Health

Health is sometimes thought to be the absence of disease. If you don't have a virus, tumor, ulcer, or some other pathology in one of the body systems, you must be healthy. We, like many health care professionals, don't care much for this notion of health: It implies that either you have health or you don't. Being healthy involves more than not being sick. An important part of health is physical well-being. Being happy, feeling fulfilled, and having a good social support network are also important. Thus we might think of health as made up of *physical*, *emotional*, and *social* components. We might also think of it as occurring on a continuum that ranges from very poor to very good. The World Health Organization has used this definition of health since the 1940s. Some people don't like this definition because it means you have to be doing well in all three of the physical, emotional, and social areas to have very good health. This may not always be possible, but it's something we can all try to achieve.

Anxiety

Think back to times when you've felt anxious about something other than your health. Did you feel you were in danger? Were you uncertain about what might happen? Did you feel distressed?

Anxiety occurs when you *think* something bad is going to happen but you are *uncertain* that it will. For example, in preparing to give a speech, you may begin to feel anxious as you wonder whether it will go over well with the audience. Or, while taking a short cut through an unfamiliar neighborhood, you might begin to worry about whether some shady character is going to pull you into a back lane and mug you. The anticipation of harm, combined with uncertainty about how threatening the situation will actually be, creates feelings of uneasiness and apprehension—those vague feelings that something may be wrong or that something terrible might happen.

But anxiety is not simply a feeling of uneasiness or apprehension. It also involves changes in our physiology and behavior. When we're anxious, our body responds in ways designed to prepare us to take action against potential threats: heart rate quickens, muscles tense, breathing becomes labored, and we might sweat, feel nauseated, and experience other bodily changes. Because the source of the threat isn't clear, the best action to take usually isn't obvious. In other words, it's difficult to know what to do or how best to respond in the anxiety-provoking circumstance. This uncertainty also sometimes carries over into our daily lives. In our speech example, the anxiety over doing a good job during the speech may actually prevent good performance. Why? Because you may spend too much time worrying about possible outcomes rather than rehearsing and doing other things that contribute to success.

Anxiety is similar to but not the same as fear. Fear is an emotional response that occurs when you're confronted with a *specific* threatening situation or object. If a shady character did pull you into a back lane while holding a knife to your throat, you would be feeling fear, not anxiety, because you know exactly what is threatening you! Likewise, if you are hiking and come face-to-face with a grizzly bear, you're not uncertain about the danger.

Anxiety and fear can be important in helping us get by in our environment and perform at our best. Our daily lives are filled with situations in which that extra jolt of adrenaline helps us deal with a challenge. Without some degree of fear, you would be very unlikely to even attempt to escape that grizzly bear! Nor would we perform at our best during a job interview or on a test. Consider our speech example again. A person with a moderate degree of anxiety about speaking to a large audience is likely to be well prepared—knowing her material, taking along a few jokes to break the ice, and having handy a few visual props to keep the audience's attention—whereas a person with little or no anxiety may go in unprepared and have to wing it. But for those in whom anxiety can be excessive, the feelings of uncertainty and apprehension may by very intense, may last for long periods of time, and may go way beyond being a helpful response. A person who is too anxious about giving a speech may freeze up and be unable to speak in front of the audience or, more likely, might not even show up to talk at all. Unfortunately, many people experience so much anxiety that it interferes with their ability to manage their day-to-day living—their relationships suffer, they miss work, they feel depressed, and they don't know how to make it stop. Recent statistics indicate that anxiety disorders have surpassed depression as the most common mental health problem experienced by North Americans.

Health Anxiety

If we put together the individual definitions of *health* and *anxiety*, we get the following: Health anxiety is the feeling that your physical well-being, or disease-free state, is threatened and you don't know what the cause or what the outcome will be. Like other forms of anxiety, health anxiety involves changes in thoughts, physiology, and behavior. Also like other forms of anxiety, health anxiety can range from mild to severe. Mild health anxiety can be temporary and can sometimes be a signal to follow up on some bodily change or sensation by seeking advice from a doctor. But it can also be excessive and preoccupying, as in the examples of Joan, Jonathan, and Bob. When health anxiety is out of proportion to the risk of disease and persists even though there is no evidence of disease, mental health professionals often refer to it as a health anxiety disorder. Like the other anxiety disorders, it has an impact on all aspects of health. The trick, of course, lies in figuring out what is out of proportion and inappropriately persistent. That is, how much is too much?

Are Your Bodily Sensations Imagined or Real?

The bodily sensations or concerns you're experiencing are real—very real. Any sane person would worry about a headache that doesn't go away or about waking up with a stomachache every morning. The trouble is that these are not always signals of disease—in fact, they rarely are—and the worry can grow out of proportion to the actual threat.

Where do the bothersome bodily sensations come from? They might arise from changes to your diet, activity levels and preferences, or sleeping habits. For example, if burritos are not something you regularly eat, you may experience some stomach upset after having a few of them (especially if you use extra hot sauce). Also a number of *minor* physical ailments can have signs and symptoms that may look like a more serious condition. Lumps in the breast may be benign (harmless) fibroids rather than cancerous tumors, clumsiness may be due to fatigue and not multiple sclerosis, and headache may be the result of a stressful day rather than a blood clot in the brain. In many cases, the sensations are part of the body's anxiety response. Anxiety is associated with many bodily changes and sensations, including shortness of breath, pounding or racing heart, chest tightness, muscle tension, fatigue, dizziness, stomach upset (for example, nausea, bloating), diarrhea, flushing or hot flashes, and trembling or shakiness.

These sensations, whether they come from changes in your lifestyle, minor physical ailments, or anxiety, have one thing in common: They are harmless. But if you notice these changes and start to worry about whether they are signaling disease, you are very likely to become more anxious, and the changes will persist and possibly get worse. One of the main goals of this book is to show you how to identify and effectively respond to your health anxiety before it spirals out of proportion to the point where it actually perpetuates the very sensations that cause you concern.

The Health Anxiety Cycle

To successfully deal with excessive health anxiety, you need to learn how to determine whether bothersome bodily sensations and symptoms are harmless. Visiting a doctor is a good (and essential) first step. Some health-related worries may be associated with health issues that your doctor should look at. Bodily sensations such as stomach upset or a pounding heart or feelings such as being off balance and clumsy can happen for any number of reasons. It's important to figure out as soon as possible whether they're related to a disease so that proper medical care can be given. Quite often the doctor is able to figure out the cause of the sensations and make a recommendation that leads to relief. For example, Jeff went to see his doctor after having had a headache for five days for which Tylenol provided no relief. The doctor determined that Jeff had a bacterial sinus infection and prescribed an antibiotic that relieved the headaches within two days. The positive outcome of Jeff's visit to his doctor, though, may not represent your typical experience when visiting your physician.

If the doctor rules out physical disease, then seeking alternate explanations is the next step. Unfortunately, many people with health anxiety get stuck at Step 1, visiting their doctors repeatedly or seeking the opinions of many doctors and specialists. Have you visited your doctor several times in a short period of time about the same health concern? Have you visited several doctors in the hope that one would give you a physical explanation for your health concern? The habit of repeatedly visiting doctors for the same concern can provide reassurance that you're okay. But that feeling of reassurance is short-lived and can prolong rather than help resolve the health anxiety.

Sarah: "My doctor thinks I'm a crock."

Sarah went to see her doctor again yesterday because she was very concerned that a new lump in her breast was cancerous. Her doctor said, "Sarah, there's no indication that the lumps in your breast are cancerous. I want you to stop worrying so much about your health. You've been to see me at least 12 times over the past seven or eight months, and I've sent you for many tests. Each time the tests have come back negative. Sarah, there's simply nothing seriously wrong with you."

Sarah was apologetic about repeatedly checking with the doctor to see if her breast lumps were cancerous. "I'm sorry for pestering you, doctor, but I just can't stop worrying that I've got breast cancer. It runs in my family. My mother, one of my aunts, and my grandmother all died of breast cancer when they were about my age." Her doctor again reassured her that nothing was wrong. Sarah left the office feeling somewhat better, but by the time she arrived home she was once again worried and upset. She liked her doctor but was beginning to feel that he was incompetent and, for certain, wasn't taking her concerns seriously.

What if the mammograms and blood tests had simply failed to detect cancer? Sarah had heard on the news that this happened all the time. "Maybe we should try to get an appointment at the Mayo Clinic," she said to her husband. "Jennifer was telling me that someone she knew had gone to the Mayo and that they found that he did have cancer even though his own doctors said there wasn't anything wrong with him." Her husband suggested she just listen to her doctor and not worry so much. Sarah tried to sleep that night but couldn't. Just before going to bed, she examined her breasts, noting that they were very painful and that several lumps seemed to have grown larger. "My God, I'm going to die just like Mom, and nobody seems to care. My doctor thinks I'm a crock and my husband is starting to think I'm crazy."

Sarah's interaction with her doctor is quite common. She repeatedly visited her doctor over concerns about cancer. Numerous tests ordered by the doctor failed to reveal evidence of physical disease. In an effort to comfort Sarah, and perhaps to get her to stop visiting so often, her doctor told her nothing was wrong with her. This reassurance was helpful only for a short period of time. Soon after, Sarah was questioning the competence of her doctor and wondering whether she should seek another opinion. She also became increasingly concerned about the lumps in her breasts, checking them 10 to 20 times per day on average, and felt that nobody, including her husband, understood what she was going through. Her desire to visit the Mayo Clinic, despite not being able to afford it, began to cause strife in her relationship with her husband. As she lost confidence in her doctor, Sarah began visiting other doctors, one of whom was familiar with health anxiety and referred her to us.

We assured Sarah that we understood her breast lumps were real and that they were affecting her life. We asked her a number of questions, many of which we will have you ask yourself toward the end of this chapter. Based on her answers to our questions, combined with information from her medical history, we concluded that Sarah had one of the several health anxiety disorders experienced by millions of North Americans.

We began our work with Sarah by having her consider how her specific type of health anxiety might be contributing to swollen and painful breast lumps. She was, as expected, skeptical at first. But as we had her consider alternatives—such as whether she believed it was possible that the swelling and pain might be due to palpating her breasts every hour on the hour all day long—her interest in learning more about the health anxiety disorders and about how she might test whether some of our strategies would alleviate some of her symptoms increased. Sarah turned the corner toward recovery once she grasped that the underlying nature of her condition could be explained by something other than physical disease. Let's see whether the problems that brought you to this book resemble any of the health anxiety disorders described in the next section.

Common Health Anxiety Disorders

Health anxiety can range from very mild to very severe. Severe forms of health anxiety differ from milder forms in the amount of emotional upset and the disruption they create in the activities of day-to-day living and relationships with others. More severe forms cause greater distress and more difficulties at work and home. After a specialist ruled out any problems with his eyes, Barry wondered whether recent episodes of blurred vision might be related to a brain tumor. Aside from mentioning his concerns to his girlfriend and spending a few minutes each day thinking about it, his life remained pretty much unaffected. Sarah, on the other hand, was feeling more and more abandoned by her husband and friends as she became increasingly convinced she had breast cancer. Stan, concerned that he might have contracted a serious skin disease, spent so much time picking at every little blemish he could find on his body that he was unable to get any of his work done and is now failing his night course. He knows he spends too much time picking at and prodding his body, but he just can't stop, and his skin is now a mess, with scabs all over. These examples represent the most common health anxiety disorders, which fall under the categories of hypochondriasis, disease phobia, and somatic delusions.

Hypochondriasis

The American Psychiatric Association's *Diagnostic and Statistical Manual of Mental Disorders*, now in its revised fourth edition (DSM-IV-TR), classifies hypochondriasis as a somatoform disorder. This is a group of disorders characterized by physical symptoms that suggest some sort of general medical condition (or disease) but that aren't completely expained by the disease. Hypochondriasis is defined as "the preoccupation with the fear of having, or the idea that one has, a serious disease based on the person's misinterpretation of bodily symptoms or bodily functions" (p. 485). Although DSM-IV-TR classifies it differently, we find it useful to consider hypochondriasis a health anxiety disorder because anxiety and worry are such predominant features. Hypochondriasis also shares a number of characteristics with other anxiety disorders, in particular panic disorder, generalized anxiety disorder, and obsessive-compulsive disorders, discussed further in Chapter 3.

In determining whether you have hypochondriasis, a cognitive-behavioral therapist may ask questions about disease-related worry, as well as questions about the way you perceive and interpret bodily sensations and symptoms. For example, we asked Sarah questions such as "Is your health on your mind a lot?" "Do you worry a lot about getting sick or being ill?" and "What symptoms do you have and why do you think they indicate that you have a disease?" You might also be asked about:

- Your medical history and history of medical tests,
- The degree to which you're convinced that your symptoms are physical,
- The amount of distress you experience when thinking about your bodily sensations,
- Limitations in your social, occupational, and leisure activities,
- The duration of your symptoms, and
- Emotional difficulties you may be experiencing.

Sarah's mind was constantly buzzing with thoughts about the lumps in her breasts being cancerous, about the fact that she was being a pest to her doctor, that she might die, and that her doctor and loved ones thought she was going crazy. Physically she felt "keyed up" much of the time and most recently was having trouble sleeping. Although she could still function reasonably well at her job, she was spending increasing amounts of time examining her breasts for changes and new lumps, and her relationship with her husband was deteriorating. She also was seeking reassurance from her doctor, her husband, and, most recently, her children with increasing frequency. Sarah was diagnosed with hypochondriasis.

Disease Phobia

Disease phobia is a type of specific phobia (fears that focus on one or a very few things, such as spiders or heights), an anxiety disorder associated with fear of contracting or ultimately dying of one or more *specific* diseases. For example, a person may fear developing multiple sclerosis or contracting some form of contagious disease. Bob, who goes to great lengths to avoid germs, has disease phobia. Those with disease phobia don't typically believe they already have the disease, and, as a consequence, they don't exhibit the bodily sensations and symptoms associated with the disease they fear. They do, however, have considerable anxiety, and they may experience muscle tension, lightheadedness, difficulty breathing, and racing heart. Also, they may avoid places or situations associated with the disease they fear. Not only did Bob start wearing latex gloves to avoid direct contact with germs, but soon after he also refused to use public washrooms, even in the most urgent circumstances. His willingness to have bladder and bowel movements only in his bathroom at home resulted in unexpected absences from work and unexplained early departures from leisure and social activities.

Mike: "I don't want to catch SARS."

Although he lived in a small rural town and had not traveled for the past two or three years, Mike was afraid he was going to contract SARS. His fear continued to escalate, and for four weeks he left his home infrequently. When he did go out, he wore a surgical mask and latex gloves and did whatever he could to avoid people. Whenever he was in close proximity to another person, his heart began to race, he became sweaty, and he felt that he had to "get out of there." When a friend from Toronto called to say that he was in town to see his family, Mike made several excuses to ensure that a visit was not possible. Although he recognized that these sorts of measures were extreme, he wanted to do everything possible to avoid contracting SARS.

In determining whether you have disease phobia, a cognitive-behavioral therapist may ask questions regarding your fears about contracting a serious disease, such as "Are you concerned that you might catch a serious disease?" and "Do you get panicky whenever you see things like sick people or hospitals, or hear news about viruses?" They might also ask questions about:

- Your degree of fear relative to other people,
- Things you avoid because of your fear,
- Limitations in your social, occupational, and leisure activities, and
- Your level of distress.

Somatic Delusions

Some people's beliefs about having a serious disease are so strong and unshakable that they are considered delusional. Generally speaking, delusions are erroneous beliefs, based on some sort of misinterpretation of perceptions or experiences, that are held with conviction and near absolute certainty. The most common forms of delusions regarding the idea that the body is diseased, sickly, or not functioning properly are that:

- One is emitting a foul odor from the skin or opening into the body, such as the mouth or rectum,
- One is infested with insects or parasites,
- Parts of the body are misshapen or ugly, despite objective evidence to the contrary, and
- Parts of the body, such as the circulatory system or bowels, are not working properly.

Vicky: "People don't like me because I smell bad."

For the past five years Vicky has held a strong belief that she emits a foul odor during menstruation. She describes the odor as a "mixture of blood, urine, and rotting flesh." She had her first period early, at age 10, and was teased by her schoolmates. Vicky attributes the teasing to "smelling bad." Now 15 years old, she rarely leaves the house except to attend classes, has never had a boyfriend, and has no girlfriends. She is certain that her extraordinary efforts to stay clean and mask body odor during her menstrual periods—showering at least six times a day and using a can of body spray daily—are entirely ineffective.

A mental health professional may ask a variety of questions regarding the nature of disease-related beliefs and convictions, such as "Are parts of your body malfunctioning?" and "Is your body occupied by parasites?" when determining whether you have somatic delusions. In many respects, people with somatic delusions are similar to those with hypochondriasis. The primary difference is in the degree to which people with these conditions understand that their concerns over having a disease or bodily malfunction are excessive or unreasonable. Those with hypochondriasis, like Sarah, understand this to some degree; those with somatic delusions, like Vicky, understand it less if at all.

The Challenge

You still may not want to think that anxiety or aspects of your lifestyle, not physical disease, are responsible for your physical concerns. But, as we discussed earlier, it's a possibility. Remember that health anxiety can range from very mild to very severe; every person is unique. One of the primary challenges we face when assessing a person in our research and clinical work is determining where the person falls on the continuum. Does a person have too much health anxiety? Experience with a lot of people with health anxiety disorders helps us make this judgment. You have more experience with your own symptoms than anybody else, and so you can do the same.

How Much Is Too Much?

To answer the question, How much health anxiety is too much? you must answer a number of other questions that have to do with specific aspects of your worry and the ways in which it affects your ability to carry out your day-to-day routine. Ask yourself the following questions:

1. How much time do I spend worrying that I have or might contract a disease?
2. How often have I visited my doctor about the same symptoms despite her reassurances that there's nothing physically wrong?
3. How much time am I spending checking the Internet and other sources of disease information, and in what ways is that interfering with my ability to get other things done?
4. Have I stopped doing anything that I enjoy because of my beliefs that I'm sick or might catch a disease?
5. To what extent are my worries interfering with my ability to work?

If your answer to question 1 was, in so many words, *pretty often*; if you've consulted your doctor several times about the same thing despite no evidence of anything wrong; and if you can see that you're spending so much time and emotional energy on worrying about your health that your house is a mess, your relationships languishing, your hobbies abandoned, and your work suffering, health anxiety is probably a significant negative factor in your life. Let's take a closer look, using a well-established test of health anxiety.

Over the years a number of tests have been developed to assist researchers and doctors in evaluating patients for health anxiety. We've found that the Whiteley Index, printed on the next page, is particularly useful for self-assessment, and we suggest you complete it now.

Give yourself a point for every *yes* response to all questions except number 9, for which you get a point if you circled *no*. This should produce a score between 0 and 14. Higher scores indicate higher levels of health anxiety. A score of 8 or more usually indicates a high probability of a health anxiety disorder.

If you scored near 8 or higher, and if this high score is consistent with your responses to the previous list of five questions, try finishing this book and using the techniques offered as self-help. If you haven't done so already, we also strongly recommend that you raise and discuss the issue of health anxiety with your doctor. If you feel you need help approaching your doctor about this, you'll find useful guidelines for doing so in the last section of this book. Please keep in mind that if your problem seems to be on the more severe end of the continuum, only an evaluation by an experienced clinician can confirm that you have a health anxiety disorder and rule out the possibility that your high score is not due to depression or another emotional disorder (discussed later in this book).

How This Book Can Help

If you believe your health anxiety is excessive and causing you harm at some level, you can move on to Chapter 2 for a more in-depth explanation of how people come to explain (or form certain beliefs about) the bodily sensations they experience and, importantly, how anxiety can influence both the explanations and the sensations experienced. Here we provide you with the building blocks for learning strategies that will help you change the way you think about and respond to the bodily sensations that you are now interpreting as disease related. Chapters 3 and 4 focus on other mental health conditions, including the anxiety disorders and depression, which often co-occur with excessive health anxiety. You'll learn the relationship between health anxiety and these other conditions, as well as methods you can use to self-assess anxiety and mood disorders. You need to be frank about how much problems with other types of anxiety or depressed mood are affecting you because, ultimately, these will affect the way you'll approach helping yourself overcome your health worries.

You may be so focused on your body that it's hard to believe the key to better health may be in your thoughts and actions. In the second section of this book, "Breaking the Health Anxiety Cycle," we outline strategies that you can use to *get on with living life*. Stress is a fact of life, but that doesn't mean you can't learn to relax. Chapter 5 teaches you exercises you can use to relax in any situa-

The Whiteley Index

Here are some questions about your health. Circle either YES or NO to indicate your answer to each question.

1. Do you often worry about the possibility that you have got a serious illness?   **YES**   NO

2. Are you bothered by many pains and aches?   **YES**   NO

3. Do you find that you are often aware of various things happening in your body?   **YES**   NO

4. Do you worry a lot about your health?   **YES**   NO

5. Do you often have the symptoms of very serious illness?   **YES**   NO

6. If a disease is brought to your attention (through the radio, television, newspapers, or someone you know) do you worry about getting it yourself?   **YES**   NO

7. If you feel ill and someone tells you that you are looking better, do you become annoyed?   YES   **NO**

8. Do you find that you are bothered by many different symptoms?   **YES**   NO

9. Is it easy for you to forget about yourself, and think about all sorts of other things?   YES   **NO**

10. Is it hard for you to believe the doctor when he or she tells you there is nothing for you to worry about?   YES   **NO**

11. Do you get the feeling that people are not taking your illness seriously enough?   YES   **NO**

12. Do you think that you worry about your health more than most people?   **YES**   NO

13. Do you think there is something seriously wrong with your body?   **YES**   NO

14. Are you afraid of illness?   **YES**   NO

Note. Score 1 point for every YES circled, except for question 9 where 1 point is scored for circling NO. Reprinted with kind permission from Professor Issy Pilowsky, Department of Psychiatry, University of Adelaide, South Australia 5001, Australia.

tion. People who are so focused on their health worries often overlook many other things that contribute to their stress. So you will also learn effective relaxation techniques for alleviating stress that arises from daily hassles and the generally hectic world we live in. In Chapter 6 you'll learn to change those patterns of thought that are feeding your health anxiety, replacing them with ones that feed good health. No, it's not "all in your head," but we all have unhelpful patterns of thinking that influence the way we feel and behave. Chapter 7 will equip you with ways for changing behaviors that feed your health anxiety and keep it alive.

By the time you get to the final section of the book, "Maintaining Your Gains," you should be well on your way to getting your worries about health under control. But what about other people? The final chapters of this book are meant to help you provide others—your doctor, your family, your friends—with practical advice on the most effective ways of helping you deal with and overcome your health anxiety. People with health anxiety are often told by their doctors that they're simply "worrying too much over nothing." This isn't helpful. In Chapter 8 we outline the steps you can take to improve interactions with your doctor and to help your doctor help you. We also provide practical decision rules to help you determine when you should visit your doctor. This is critical. We want you to get to the point at which you seek out medical advice only when it's absolutely essential. Chapter 9 is designed to help you help your family and friends understand what you're going through and how they can best help you manage and recover. Finally, in Chapter 10 we outline additional things you can do to get on with enjoying life, strategies for dealing with flare-ups of health anxiety, and, if needed, the types of specialized treatments that are available to you and guidelines for deciding when and how to go about getting this type of help. We've provided a number of worksheets for you to work through. You can complete them in the book or make copies from the ones at the back of the book. Now let's get started!

Two

Body and Brain
It's Not All in Your Head

Have you been told at some point, perhaps by your doctor, a friend, or a relative, that the bodily sensations that are causing you worry are "all in your head"? The implication of this message is that the things you experience in your body are imagined rather than real. This message is false. We all experience bodily sensations on a daily basis, and sometimes we wonder why they're occurring. A pounding or racing heart. Shakiness. Throbbing temples. Tingling in the ribcage. Chills. Dizziness. Stomach pain and discomfort. Heavy, aching limbs. These sensations are real—all too real—and can occur for any number of reasons. Sometimes they're the harmless expressions of a properly functioning and healthy body, sometimes they're symptoms of common minor ailments, and less often they're symptoms of a serious medical condition. Quite often, though, people with health anxiety *misinterpret* bodily sensations; that is, they believe these sensations are signals of disease when they aren't.

In this chapter we consider the causes of bodily sensations. We also look at ways that you may have tried to understand these sensations—the personal theories you've developed to explain them—and the path you took to arrive at the belief that the sensations you experience are symptomatic of disease. By understanding the ways you came to the conclusion that harmless sensations indicate that your health is in jeopardy, you'll be able to uncover paths to other explanations.

Why Do Bodily Sensations Occur?

The human body, much like a refrigerator or automobile, can be noisy at times. And it can be noisy even when working properly. But where does the noise—

these unwanted bodily sensations—come from, and why does it occur? There are many different sources and reasons. For example, noise can arise from disruptions to the typical day-to-day functioning of your body, such as might occur from changes in your diet, activity levels, or sleeping habits. It can also arise as a consequence of:

- Prolonged inactivity,
- Symptoms of *minor* ailments, or
- Arousal associated with fear, anxiety, and other emotions.

Let's take a closer look at these sources of bodily sensations.

Changes in Routine

Many of us have a typical daily pattern of activity that we follow without much deviation. We go to bed at the same time every night, get up at the same time every morning, go through the same series of steps in getting ourselves or loved ones ready for the day, take the same route to work, and so on. However, in today's world, it's not uncommon for our routines to be disrupted at times. This can happen intentionally, such as when we decide to become more active and start exercising on a regular basis. It can also occur unexpectedly. For example, you may get stuck in a traffic jam that delays your getting home, or you might have a night when despite your best efforts you simply can't sleep well. Whether intentional or unexpected, changes to routine can trigger a number of bodily changes, *even in people who are healthy.*

Think about the last time you slept poorly. How did you feel the next day? In addition to being tired, did you feel shaky, have achy, painful, and tense muscles, and eyes that seemed dry and blurry? Perhaps you felt a number of other bodily sensations as well. Headachy? Sluggish? Detached from things? It's not unusual to feel these things following poor sleep. Similarly, changes in activity, such as exercise or overexertion, can promote immediately noticeable increases in heart rate and breathing rate during activity, hunger pangs and stomach activity shortly after, and muscle tenderness, aching, and shakiness in the hours and days that follow.

There are, in fact, an almost endless number of changes in routine that can promote noise in your body. Short-term changes to your diet can induce mild hypoglycemia (low blood sugar levels) that, in turn, can produce faintness, sweating, and increased heart rate. Going quickly from a sitting to standing position can lead to temporary dizziness as the result of rapid changes in blood pressure. Exposure to cold can lead to shivering and numbness, whereas too much heat can induce sweating, thirst, lightheadedness, and headache. Consuming alcohol or marijuana can induce a variety of sensations, as can spinning in circles or riding on a roller coaster. The critical issue is whether the bodily noise resulting from changes to your typical routine is indicative of an impending threat to your well-being. If you don't recognize that there are many possible harmless causes of these bodily sensations, you might mistakenly conclude that the sensations are signs of some serious disease.

Inactivity

Being inactive over a period of months, or sometimes even just a few days, is associated with poor cardiovascular fitness, muscle weakness, and fatigue. Some of the most common sensations experienced by somebody who is out of shape are:

- Shortness of breath,
- Pounding or racing heart,
- Muscle aches and pains, and
- General feelings of fatigue and tiredness.

When an inactive person resumes a more active lifestyle, he or she will, as described earlier, experience a number or immediate and short-lived bodily sensations as a result of these altered routines.

Inactivity can also influence bodily sensations in other ways. Transient (or temporary) inactivity in an otherwise active person can produce a number of sensations. Most of us have, for example, experienced "numb bum" after sitting for lengthy periods during a long movie or lengthy road trip. Likewise, prolonged and continuing inactivity in an inactive person can lead to bodily noise. Forty-one-year-old Bill, a computer programmer, typically spent eight hours a day at his computer, rushed home to help prepare dinner and put the children to bed, and relaxed for several hours in front of the TV before going to bed. As a result of his inactivity at work and during leisure time, Bill experienced persistent low back and neck pain, as well as a general feeling of fatigue. Bill's concern was that the sensations of pain in his back and neck muscles were the result of Lou Gehrig's disease and that he would soon become immobile and, shortly thereafter, die. He hadn't even considered the possibility that his general inactivity could have something to do with these worrisome sensations.

Minor Ailments

Many minor ailments can produce unpleasant bodily sensations. For example, stomach upset can lead to bowel cramping, constipation, bloating, and pressure. In some cases, stomach upset can also cause sensations of chest tightness or pain. So can minor straining of the intercostal muscles (the muscles between the ribs). Likewise, dyspepsia, or heartburn, can lead to chest pain, burning sensations in the upper gastrointestinal tract, and feelings of nausea. Allergies can make one's inner chest and ribs feel "scratchy" or "tingly" and produce considerable congestion and pressure in the head (making it feel like it could explode) and shortness of breath, and they often cause episodes of coughing or sneezing. Diarrhea can produce discomfort and sensations of burning in the anal region. In Table 1 we've listed some of the more common minor ailments that people experience and the bodily sensations that they produce. This list is by no means complete, but it illustrates the many sensations that are associated with these conditions. Keep in mind that, although these sensations are bothersome, they are *generally harmless*. That is, they don't generally produce serious adverse effects on physical health or death.

Anxiety and Other Emotions

The human body is designed to maintain *homeostasis*, or balance, in its many functions. This balance is achieved, in part, through the operation of a specific part of the human nervous system called the autonomic nervous system, which is divided into the parasympathetic division and the sympathetic division. Each division has a different effect on the functions of many organs and muscles of the body. (A third part of the autonomic nervous system, called the enteric nervous system, meaning "gut brain," supplies the nerves to the gastrointestinal tract, pancreas, and gall bladder.) Generally speaking, the operation of the autonomic nervous system is beyond our control. It is involuntary and reflexive and is not something that we notice during a typical day. Table 2 shows the two main divisions of the autonomic nervous system and their effects on various body systems.

The parasympathetic division operates during periods of what we might call "business as usual," keeping the body functioning in a relaxed and balanced

TABLE 1. Common Ailments and the Bodily Sensations They Produce

Ailment	Typical sensation(s)
Headache	Head pain, throbbing, blurry vision
Cough/cold	Sore threat, chest tightness
Diarrhea	Stomach and intestinal pain, cramping, burning
Skin problems	Itching
Muscle soreness	Aching, heaviness, stabbing or shooting pains
Sinus congestion	Head pain, pressure, throbbing, difficulty breathing
Heartburn	Chest pain, burning in gastrointestinal tract, nausea
Menstrual cramps	Abdominal pain, low back pain, bloating
Allergies	Swelling, itching, head pressure, shortness of breath

TABLE 2. Body Systems and Structures Affected by the Parasympathetic and Sympathetic Divisions of the Autonomic Nervous System

Body system	Parasympathetic effect	Sympathetic effect
Pupil	Constriction	Dilation
Salivary glands	Increased saliva production (moist mouth)	Decreased saliva production (dry mouth)
Mucosa (oral and nasal)	Increased mucus production (moist mouth and nasal cavity)	Decreased mucus production (dry mouth and nasal cavity)
Heart	Decreased rate and contractile force	Increased rate and contractile force
Larynx, trachea, bronchi, and lungs	Contracted (slow breathing)	Relaxed (rapid breathing)
Stomach and small intestine	Increased digestive processes	Decreased digestive processes
Adrenal gland		Secretion of epinephrine and norepinephrine
Large intestine	Increased movement	Decreased movement
Kidney	Increased urine secretion	Decreased urine secretion
Bladder	Contracted and sphincter relaxed	Relaxed and sphincter closed
Liver		Increased conversion of glycogen to glucose (increased energy supply)

state. The heart beats at an average rate, breathing is steady and unlabored, and digestive processes are active. The sympathetic division, on the other hand, is activated during times of excitement and stress. The classic example of the operation of the sympathetic division is the "fight or flight" response. Recall the example in Chapter 1 of being pulled into an alley by a mugger. In this situation, your sympathetic nervous system is called into action in order to support your efforts to survive, whether that involves running away or fighting back. What happens?

- Your blood pressure increases.
- Your heart pumps more rapidly.
- Blood is restricted from flowing to your arms and legs.
- Your breathing rate increases.
- Digestive processes are put on hold.
- You feel *keyed up* and are prepared to defend yourself or flee from the mugger.

This type of bodily activation occurs not only in response to fear-provoking situations, such as facing a mugger, but also to such things as changes in room temperature, anxiety, surprise, and pain. Note the number of different bodily systems that are affected by changes in autonomic nervous system functioning. Most of these systems produce certain "noises" in the body when influenced by one of the autonomic nervous system divisions. These noises, although part and parcel of a properly functioning body, are often misinterpreted by people with health anxiety as being part of a serious disease. Stan, for example, felt his heart pound and became short of breath every time he played baseball. Although he had been an active person his whole life, and despite having passed a treadmill test that his doctor used to evaluate his heart, he worried that his heart was weak and that he would have a heart attack. He hadn't considered that his body was reacting to the excitement he felt when playing ball.

Trying to Understand Bodily Sensations: Symptom of Disease or Not?

Bodily sensations trigger thoughts that help us determine whether the feeling signals a threat to our well-being and whether we need to respond to it in order to minimize harm to our health and disruption to our daily activities (for example, by seeking our doctor's opinion). What's causing this sensation? we ask ourselves, consciously or unconsciously. Is it a result of an injury or disease? Should I report the sensation to my doctor and have it checked out?

On Signs and Symptoms

A bodily sensation that's perceived as being unpleasant and assumed to be a consequence of a disease is referred to as a *symptom*. This means that all the sensations we discussed as possible products of a healthy and properly functioning body can be referred to as symptoms under certain circumstances. Sensations are considered symptoms when they:

- Are perceived as being troublesome and cause disruption to your daily activities,
- Are believed to have some link to disease, and
- Lead to self-care (for example, resting, taking over-the-counter medications) or seeking advice from a health care professional.

The symptoms you experience can't be seen or felt by others. They're subjective, and thus the only way they can be understood by another person, such as your doctor, is through your description of what you are feeling in your body. Think about the last time you experienced pain. How did you let others know about it?

You couldn't show them your pain, so you probably tried to describe it to them. "It hurts so bad. It feels like someone has split my head open with an axe and pierced my eyes with ice picks." Contrast this to a *sign*. A sign is an easily observed marker of possible injury or pathology. For example, swelling around the ankle after one has fallen is a sign that some part of the ankle, perhaps ligaments or tendons, may be damaged. An increase in the number of a particular type of white blood cell is a sign that cancer may be present. Despite differences between symptoms and signs—symptoms being subjective and signs directly observable—both are real experiences.

You may be concerned with both signs and symptoms. It's the symptoms, however, that most people with health anxiety find most bothersome and concerning. Why? Symptoms are a reflection of (1) your perception of what is going on in your body and (2) your interpretation of the importance of this to your health and well-being. Symptoms, by definition, occur when the body produces sensations that we believe to be out of place. So any noise in your body is a symptom of disease if you believe it is caused by disease. But the presence of symptoms doesn't equal the presence of disease. Similarly, signs of disease don't equal the presence of disease. Recall Sarah, introduced in Chapter 1. The lumps in her breasts were signs that cancer might be present. It wasn't. The lumps were benign (harmless) fibrous tissue that many women develop as they grow older. This type of misinterpretation—thinking that bodily sensations and observable signs of possible disease *are* disease—is very common. This is true for all of us, but particularly so for people with a lot of health anxiety.

(Mis)Interpreting Signs and Symptoms

In trying to understand the signs and symptoms we experience, we go through a process similar to that of any trained medical doctor diagnosing a patient. We first collect information about the symptom:

- When did it begin?
- How much discomfort is there?
- Does it get better or worse under certain conditions or at certain times?

These data are then used to make a tentative diagnosis. Most of us go through this process before arriving at the doctor's office and, as a result, have our own idea of what might be wrong. We might consult family and friends for their opinions ("What do you think it is?" "Based on what I have told you, do you think I might have a brain tumor?") and seek advice on actions to be taken.

Our tentative diagnosis is typically placed in the context of what we know and have learned about disease. This means that our past history with disease, our understanding of disease processes, and societal influences on what symptoms mean and on how we report them all have an impact on the way we interpret our signs and symptoms. For example, growing up we learn that certain sensations are associated with certain conditions and that these conditions have consequences and methods of treatment. Consider throbbing in the right temple. What does this symptom typically indicate? What are its consequences and how might the symptom be relieved? Most people associate this particular symptom with a diagnosis of *headache*. We've learned through personal experience, or from observing a parent or sibling, that headaches place limits on the things we do when we have one. What we've learned will also influence whether we rest, take an over-the-counter painkiller, or visit the doctor to get relief from the headache. However, if your father told you he was having throbbing in the right temple just prior to having a stroke, you may respond to throbbing in your head quite differently. You may think, "Oh my, it's happening to me too!" The bottom line is that our experiences shape the way we interpret and, in some cases, misinterpret noise in our bodies.

Let's look at the possible outcomes that exist between symptom interpretation and disease. As shown in Figure 1, there are four possibilities. These include (1) hits, (2) misses, (3) correct rejections, and (4) false alarms. *Hits* occur when a person reports a symptom that is related to an identifiable disease process. For example, a hit occurred when Farley reported symptoms of faintness and radiating chest pain that were determined by his doctor to result from coronary artery disease. In this case, the symptoms indicated disease. A *miss* would have occurred had he not reported his symptoms, preferring to wait until the next week to do so or believing them to be due to passing indigestion despite actually having a disease. *Correct rejections* occur when a person chooses to manage his or her own symptoms of a minor ailment (such as chest pain and gastrointestinal irritation associated with heartburn) or when he or

	Bodily "noise" caused by serious disease	Bodily "noise" caused by minor ailment or regular body functioning
Symptom reported	Hit (serious situation correctly identified)	False alarm (minor symptoms or harmless sensations prompt worry and medical attention)
Symptom not reported	Miss (serious situation not attended to)	Correct rejection (minor symptoms or harmless sensations self-managed or ignored)

FIGURE 1. **Four possible scenarios between symptoms and disease.**

she ignores (does not attribute to disease) harmless bodily noise. *False alarms* occur when medical advice is sought for symptoms of minor ailments or bodily noise associated with the functioning of a healthy body. Had Farley's symptoms been the result of heartburn, rather than coronary artery disease, his visit to the doctor would have been a false alarm. These four possible scenarios apply to signs, as well.

Hits and correct rejections represent accurate interpretations of bodily sensations and symptoms and lead to appropriately targeted use of the health care system. Misses and false alarms, on the other hand, represent misinterpretations of bodily signs and sensations. The consequences of a miss can be severe. Had Farley chosen to ignore or put off seeking a doctor's advice regarding his symptoms of lightheadedness and chest pain, he might have suffered a heart attack. The consequences of false alarms, especially when the interpretive process that leads to them occurs repeatedly and over long periods of time, can also be serious because health anxiety is maintained at high levels and because it leads to uncalled-for use of a doctor's time. False alarms are very common in people with health anxiety.

List the signs and symptoms you've experienced in the past week or two on Worksheet 1. Try to list as many as you can. If you've had the same sign or symptom more than once during this time, list it as many times as you recall having had it. Beside each sign or symptom, indicate what you thought was wrong, how much anxiety you had, how you responded, and, if you visited a doctor about the symptom, what medical diagnosis you received. Finally, based on all the information you have at this point, make a decision as to whether each of the signs and symptoms listed represents a hit, a miss, a correct rejection, or a false alarm. You can refer back to this worksheet as we explore explanations *other than disease* for the situations in which you experienced false alarms.

Although misses and false alarms both have potentially serious consequences, the false alarms are most relevant in the context of health anxiety. Dr. Howard Leventhal, a noted authority on the psychology of symptom perception, suggests that false alarms are more likely to occur when a person is fearful or anxious about the meaning of a symptom. It shouldn't be surprising, then, that although all people are prone to having false alarms, those with health anxiety tend to have more of them. But why this is the case?

Selective Attention

People with health anxiety usually consider themselves to be especially sensitive to bodily sensations and report experiencing more pain and other unpleasant bodily sensations than people who are not anxious about their health. This has led some experts to wonder whether people with health anxiety are better than others at detecting even the slightest noises in their bodies. The research,

Worksheet 1. Symptom Interpretation Form

Day and date	Symptom	Initial thoughts	Intensity of anxiety (0–100)	Response	Medical opinion	Scenario
Example	Heart racing and shortness of breath	Believed I was having a heart attack	90	Rushed to emergency room	Nothing wrong. Likely an anxiety attack	False alarm
Example	Headache and sore eyes	Thought it might be a brain tumor but more likely a cold	25	Went to doctor the next day	Sinus infection	Hit (for the cold)
Example	Lumps in right breast	Thought I had breast cancer	99	Visited several doctors and specialists	Harmless fibroids	False alarm

although still inconclusive, doesn't provide convincing evidence for this. It could be that people with health anxiety have really noisy bodies rather than that they are more sensitive about detecting what's going on in their bodies. In other words, if you're anxious about your health, you may experience more bodily sensations—pain, aches, itching, heart palpitation, upset stomach, head pressure—than do other people.

Extra bodily noise could be related to biological factors. Very little research has been done in this area. Although differences in certain brain structures and neurotransmitters that influence bodily sensations may be important, we really don't know enough at this point to be sure of this. Another explanation that we know more about has to do with the way people with health anxiety pay attention to things.

Growing evidence shows that people with health anxiety spend too much time paying attention to their bodies. And when attention is so focused on something, we tend to notice it more. Consider, for example, the mother and father of a new baby who has just been put to sleep. Wanting to be prepared to respond when needed, they listen carefully for any noises the baby might make. They even use a baby monitor that allows them to better hear whatever happens in the baby's room. While going about other household activities they are very attentive, not only to sounds made by the baby but to *all* noises in the house. Listening for the baby, it seems, alerts them to sounds they once didn't notice—creaks in the floor, the refrigerator motor running, a flyer being dropped in the mailbox. The same thing occurs when your attention is directed inward to the functioning of your body. Look back at the symptoms you reported in Worksheet 1. Are there instances when you focused most of your attention on the symptom? Did this make the symptoms worse? Did it increase your anxiety?

The research tends to support this idea. People who report having current symptoms, as well as those who do not, report more symptoms when a researcher asks them to deliberately focus attention on their bodies. This phenomenon is rather easy to demonstrate. To do so, you can try the following: Say to a friend "I just saw a small spider crawling on my pant leg. I'm not sure where it went. I'm feeling kind of scratchy and crawly." Now watch your friend for a few minutes to see if he or she checks or scratches his or her body any more than usual. Your friend may even tell you he or she is now feeling the same way. Similarly, in our own research we've found that people with high levels of health anxiety, but not those without, selectively pay attention to words that depict disease states or outcomes—words such as *tumor*, *stroke*, *palpitations*, and *death*. These examples suggest that focusing attention on the internal functions of the body, as well as on things in the environment (such as media reports about the causes and consequences of disease), can create noise in the body that is misinterpreted as being related to disease.

Several things increase the likelihood that you'll pay close attention to your body. These include:

- The degree to which you're focused on other things,
- Other people attending to and discussing the type of sensation you're experiencing,
- A general tendency to amplify (or overstate) the discomfort associated with sensations resulting from typical body functions, and
- Your beliefs about health and sickness.

Body versus External Focus

Our ability to attend to things is limited. That is, attention is a resource that can "run out." You've likely experienced situations in which you've run out of attention, such as sitting through a very long and boring meeting or trying to listen and respond to several people who are all talking to you at the same time. If your attention is focused on a task outside of your body, you're far less likely to notice bodily sensations. We're less likely to notice "numb bum" when completely engaged by a movie. Athletes who experience injury during competition and soldiers wounded in battle often don't notice their condition until later on. Why? Because their attention is focused on things occurring outside of their bodies. On the other hand, when nothing else is grabbing your attention, you're more likely to notice bodily sensations.

Influence of Others

If other people are paying attention to bodily sensations and symptoms, you're more likely to do so as well. If you tried the "spider demonstration," you would have observed this effect. When others scratch, yawn, or cough, we're more likely to do so, particularly when there is little else going on around us. Also, news reports can draw our attention to the body and the sensations it produces. In 2003 there was a rash of media reports on bioterrorism and SARS, indicating, for example, that coughing and fever may be a sign of infection. Although these types of reports make us all vigilant toward our own coughing (and that of others) and body temperature, people with health anxiety are more likely to attribute the cough to infection from anthrax or the SARS virus. This, of course, is only one of many examples of how the media can influence your paying attention to your body and the sensations it produces. Is it possible that some of the signs and symptoms you reported in Worksheet 1 were influenced by others? For example, seeing a news piece on breast cancer or talking about a relative who recently was diagnosed with multiple sclerosis can increase the bodily sensations and symptoms you experience.

Somatic Amplification

Some people have what Dr. Arthur Barsky, a noted authority on health anxiety, has called an *amplifying somatic style*. This style is characterized by the tendency to attend to and be bothered by a wide range of bodily sensations that aren't generally related to disease. This amplifying somatic style is believed to be a trait that may be biologically based or a product of learning during the early years of childhood. Research suggests that people who have a somatic amplifying style are prone to attend to noise in their body and to be bothered by it. If you scored high on the self-test of health anxiety presented in Chapter 1 (the Whiteley Index) you may well have an amplifying somatic style.

Beliefs about Health and Sickness

This topic is so important that we'll focus on it in detail in Chapter 6. Your beliefs about the meaning of bodily sensations as they relate to health and sickness influence both the amount of attention you pay to sensations and the way you interpret them. How? As we've already pointed out, everybody experiences noise in the body, even when the body is healthy and properly functioning. But people with too much health anxiety tend to equate bodily noise with disease ("When I feel sensations is my body, it must be because I'm sick") and, conversely, the absence of bodily noise with good health ("I haven't had any bodily sensations recently, so my health must be pretty good"; "John says he's never bothered by sensations in his body; he must be super healthy"). These beliefs are helpful to some degree because they alert us that something may be wrong and that we should visit the doctor (the hits discussed earlier). However, when you believe that many or, in some cases, all bodily sensations are caused by disease, you will be focusing attention inward on these sensations, and you will have more false alarms and general anxiety about health and well-being.

The Vicious Cycle: Anxiety Revisited

We've made several important points so far:

- All people, including those who are healthy, experience noise in their bodies.
- There are many sources of bodily noise. The noise is real.
- When the noise is bothersome and prompts a desire to seek care from a health professional, it's called a symptom. Symptoms, although subjective and personal in nature, are real.
- People with health anxiety tend to focus their attention on their bodies

and seem to experience more symptoms. They continuously monitor and check their signs and symptoms.

- The signs and symptoms reported by those with health anxiety are most often not related to a disease; that is, they are false alarms.

Considering these points, it seems logical that if your doctor assures you that a sign or symptom is not related to a disease, then your concern should be resolved. For example, once the doctor determines that the persistent throbbing you reported experiencing in your right temple isn't related to stroke or a brain tumor, your worry about the throbbing should end. As you know, this isn't the case. Although your worry may decrease for a while, you soon begin checking for sensations, notice them, and, once again, interpret them as indicating that something is seriously wrong. Other sensations you notice may also cause you concern and additional worry.

Why does this persistent worry occur? We'll help you find the answer to this question. You already have some of the pieces of the puzzle. In Chapter 1 we described anxiety as an emotional reaction that occurs when you anticipate something bad happening but are uncertain that it will. In the case of health anxiety, you believe your health and well-being are threatened. The tricky thing about anxiety, particularly as it relates to perceptions of your own health, is that the anxiety itself causes numerous bodily sensations (and weakens your body to some degree, making you somewhat more susceptible to minor ailments). You might interpret these sensations of anxiety themselves as being disease related rather than as a normal body response to a situation of worry. Recall that anxiety affects the way we behave. It may increase the likelihood that we'll check our bodies for signs or symptoms of disease or that we'll avoid things that make us uncomfortable. It also affects the way we think about and interpret things ("Something terrible is going to happen"). In turn, our behaviors and thoughts can influence the physical responses within our bodies.

We often think of persistent anxiety as a vicious and nasty cycle that's self-perpetuating. A simple illustration of this cycle as it relates to health anxiety is provided in Figure 2. Your challenge, and ours, is to break this cycle. You can do this by changing the way you attend to and interpret bodily noise and by learning how to go about your daily activities in a way that promotes a sense of well-being. Look back at Worksheet 1 to the false-alarm scenario that you rated as creating the most anxiety. The sign or symptom you listed was real; it caused you concern and you sought a medical opinion. But the doctor told you that nothing was wrong. Assuming that your doctor did a thorough assessment and that disease is not responsible for your signs or symptoms, something else must be causing them. The purpose of this chapter has been to point out several alternative explanations for the signs and symptoms that lead to false alarms. Could they be a result of your being concerned about and making an honest misinterpretation

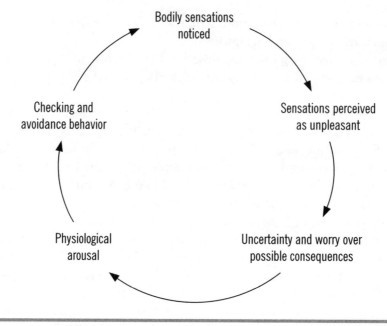

FIGURE 2. **The vicious cycle of health anxiety.**

of the noises that occur in an otherwise healthy body? Could you be stuck in the health anxiety cycle? On a scale of 0 to 10, with 0 being *not at all likely* and 10 being *very likely*, rate how likely you believe this to be possible.

If your rating was 1 or higher, then we're ready to move forward. We'll tackle the strategies for breaking the anxiety cycle in detail in the chapters of Part II. But—and this is an important *but*, so don't skip forward just yet—before learning these strategies it's important to learn about other factors that may be at play in your situation, as these may affect the way in which you'll go about breaking the anxiety cycle. Health anxiety is commonly associated with other anxiety disorders and with depressed mood. The ways in which you can assess yourself for other types of anxiety and depression and the impact they have on health anxiety are covered in detail in the following two chapters.

Three

Do I Have Some Other Anxiety Disorder?

Anxiety can be an adaptive response to situations in which the outcome is uncertain. However, when it occurs in excess, anxiety can be emotionally devastating. This type of anxiety is usually very intense, and it can last for exceedingly long periods of time (months or even years). It also creates difficulties in your relationships with friends and family and your ability to do your job. Anxiety responses that occur over and above what is needed for effective functioning (and for surviving in a world filled with uncertainty) are commonly called *anxiety disorders*.

Diagnostic criteria have been established for a number of specific anxiety disorders. We and many other therapists like to consider excessive health anxiety an anxiety disorder because it shares many characteristics with the other anxiety disorders. Technically speaking, though, it's classified as a somatoform disorder. (Recall from Chapter 1 that this is a set of disorders characterized by physical symptoms for which there is no clear medical explanation.) The major anxiety disorders described by the American Psychiatric Association in their widely used DSM-IV-TR include:

- Agoraphobia,
- Panic disorder,
- Specific phobia,
- Social phobia (or social anxiety disorder),
- Obsessive–compulsive disorder,
- Posttraumatic stress disorder,

- Acute stress disorder,
- Generalized anxiety disorder,
- Anxiety disorder due to a general medical condition, and
- Substance-induced anxiety disorder.

It's common for people with health anxiety to also have one or more of these anxiety disorders. Likewise, people who have one of these anxiety disorders often have significant health-related worries. Research has shown that panic disorder, obsessive–compulsive disorder, and generalized anxiety disorder have the most in common with health anxiety.

You may have one or more of these anxiety disorders, or you may not have any other anxiety disorder aside from your health anxiety. In this chapter we'll introduce you to several things that are important to understanding and dealing with anxiety disorders. First, we briefly describe the essential features of the three major anxiety disorders that often occur along with health anxiety. We also provide some screening questions that will allow you to determine whether you might have one of the anxiety disorders described. Second, we talk about some of the reasons that these anxiety disorders might occur at the same time as health anxiety. Finally, we wrap up the chapter with an overview of some treatment options available for panic disorder, obsessive–compulsive disorder, and generalized anxiety disorder.

Common Overlapping Anxiety Disorders

Panic Disorder

Barry: "It hit me out of the blue, like a speeding truck."

Barry, a 26-year-old photographer, went to the university health clinic after repeatedly experiencing a wildly pounding and rapidly beating heart, difficulty breathing, and light-headedness. His first attack had occurred about a year before while he was at home relaxing on the sofa: "I was feeling quite relaxed. Then, suddenly, I began feeling my heart pounding and I became very anxious. Panicky in fact. It hit me out of the blue, like a speeding truck. I had no idea what was going on, but the thought crossed my mind that I might be having a heart attack. I couldn't breathe and I felt lightheaded. It was very weird, and I felt as if I might lose control of myself." He rushed to the emergency room. Following a brief medical evaluation, he was sent home with assurances that nothing was wrong with his heart and he was just having an attack of anxiety. Over the next few weeks Barry continued having attacks spontaneously. Most of these attacks occurred during the day and, with one exception, didn't occur during sleep. The sensations were often so intense that he worried that his heart might "explode." He began avoiding many of his work assignments and had great difficulty leaving his studio for fear that he'd have another attack and lose control. When a coworker commented on the noticeable change in his work habits, Barry decided he should seek help.

A psychologist at the university health clinic assessed Barry and determined that he had panic disorder. This is an anxiety disorder characterized by abrupt and recurrent episodes of intense apprehension and fear—or panic attacks—that often occur without apparent provocation. These so-called panic attacks are very uncomfortable. They usually last for short periods and reach their peak intensity within 10 minutes. A panic attack is said to have occurred if a person experiences four or more of the 13 symptoms shown in Table 3. The term *limited symptom attack* is used to refer to panic-like episodes that have fewer than four symptoms.

To be diagnosed with panic disorder, you must have recurrent and unexpected panic attacks. That is, the attacks must *occur out of the blue* (or in the absence of any apparent danger). At least one of the unexpected panic attacks must be associated with one or more of the following:

TABLE 3. **Possible Symptoms of a Panic Attack**

1. Palpitations, pounding heart, or accelerated heart rate
2. Sweating
3. Trembling or shaking
4. Sensations of shortness of breath or smothering
5. Feelings of choking
6. Chest pain or discomfort
7. Nausea or abdominal distress
8. Feeling dizzy, unsteady, light-headed, or faint
9. Derealization (feelings of unreality) or depersonalization (being detached from yourself)
10. Fear of losing control or going crazy
11. Fear of dying
12. Paresthesias (numbness or tingling sensations)
13. Chills or hot flashes

- Persistent concern about having more attacks,
- Worry about the implications and consequences of the attacks,
- Changes in typical patterns of behavior as a result of the attacks (for example, avoidance of work or school activities).

If you panicked only when faced with a real or potentially real threat, such as coming face-to-face with a grizzly bear or thinking about taking an exam, you wouldn't be diagnosed with panic disorder. Furthermore, a doctor has to determine that your attacks aren't the result of a drug or medication or a general medical condition. For example, drinking excessive amounts of coffee or other caffeinated drinks can cause symptoms that resemble panic. So can low blood-sugar levels or an overactive thyroid gland. These need to be ruled out.

Like Barry, many people experience panic attacks for no apparent reason. In fact, somewhere between 4 and 11 percent of the population will experience an unexpected panic attack at some time in their lives. Somewhere between 1 and 2 percent will be diagnosed with panic disorder and, of these people, one-third to one-half will also develop *agoraphobia*. Agoraphobia refers to fear and avoidance of specific places or situations in which escape might be difficult (or embarrassing) if a panic attack happened. Going to a shopping mall, being in open spaces, and standing in line are commonly avoided. The onset of symptoms for many people will begin between the ages of 25 and 30, as was the case for Barry. Late adolescence is another common period for symptoms to begin (15 to 19 years). Panic disorder is diagnosed in women slightly more than twice as often as in men. If left untreated, it's usually troublesome for long periods of time (that is, it can be a chronic condition).

Several questions might help determine whether you currently have panic disorder. Ask yourself the following questions:

- Have you ever had a panic attack? (Remember that this means having an abrupt episode of intense fear or apprehension, with at least 4 of the symptoms listed in Table 3, which last for about 10 minutes.)
- Have you ever had a panic attack that has occurred unexpectedly for no apparent reason? The attack would not have been provoked by a situation or an event that caused you to be fearful (such as being mugged or witnessing a terrible accident).
- Have you had more than one unexpected panic attack?
- Do you worry a lot about having more panic attacks or that having a panic attack may harm you mentally or physically?

If you answered *yes* to all of these questions, there is a strong possibility that you have panic disorder. As we pointed out in Chapter 1, only an evaluation by an experienced doctor or mental health professional can determine whether you have an anxiety disorder. If you think you might have panic disorder, we recommend you get it checked out professionally. The symptoms of panic can cause heightened concerns about physical health and, in many cases, addressing the tendency to panic also reduces the health concerns. We describe several treatment options for panic disorder at the end of this chapter.

Obsessive–Compulsive Disorder

Martha: "The thought of them being contaminated just wouldn't go away."

Martha, a 29-year-old homemaker and mother of two toddlers, was referred by her doctor to a mental health clinic for help with feelings of depression. A psychologist completed a thorough assessment of Martha. During the assessment it came to light that she had had thoughts of suicide. But she also was having recurrent and unstoppable thoughts that she might spread germs to her children. These thoughts had become particularly noticeable since the birth of her first child, almost two years ago, and were related to Martha's belief that she was prone to bacterial infection. Her main concerns revolved around her and her children becoming infected by bacteria from contaminated food and from feces. She spent hours each day scrubbing her hands, cleaning the kitchen countertop and appliances, and disinfecting the children's eating utensils and cups. She also spent a lot of time each day washing the children after they used the washroom. "The thought of them being contaminated just wouldn't go away. So I washed everything over and over again. In the past few weeks I've spent so much time making sure that everything is germ-free that sometimes the kids have missed being fed. And their hands and faces, not to mention other parts, are starting to become dry and cracked from me scrubbing so much. Now I'm afraid that I may be as much of a threat to my kids as are the germs." Martha hadn't previously told anybody about these concerns, and she'd managed to hide her worries from her husband. She feared that he wouldn't understand.

Obsessive–compulsive disorder is an anxiety disorder that's characterized by two distinct things—obsessions and compulsions—that can occur alone or together. *Obsessions* are recurring ideas, thoughts, or impulses that intrude on the mind, are disturbing in nature, and can't be easily dismissed. Common obsessions are thoughts of being contaminated by germs, recurring doubts that you haven't locked the door, and thoughts of causing harm to loved ones. These obsessions are *not* simply excessive worries about real problems that a person is having. They are worries that don't make much sense. For example, there wasn't any compelling reason for Martha to believe that she was more likely than anyone else to carry around bacteria. *Compulsions* are repetitive behaviors that a person feels a need to perform in response to an obsession. The most common compulsions are washing, checking, and counting. These behaviors can be observable, such as repeated hand washing. They can also be mental, such as thinking a "good" thought so as to undo a "bad" thought. They're performed as a way to provide temporary relief from the feelings of anxiety. Martha's anxiety was reduced at first by scrubbing everything from countertops to her children's skin. The vast majority of people with obsessive–compulsive disorder have both obsessions and compulsions.

To be diagnosed with obsessive–compulsive disorder, you must have an obsession, a compulsion, or both. The obsession or compulsion has to create significant emotional distress, take up considerable amounts of time (an hour or more daily), or disrupt your ability to work or function properly in social situations. At some point during the disorder, you have to realize that the obsession or compulsion is excessive or unreasonable. When Martha noticed that washing was making her children's skin dry and cracking and causing them discomfort, she turned the corner to recognizing that her worries about bacteria were a bit much. Finally, as with panic disorder, a doctor needs to determine that the obsessions or compulsions aren't due to a drug or medication that you're using or to a general medical condition that you may have.

Martha is one of the approximate 2 to 3 percent of the population who will experience significant obsessions or compulsions during their lives. The symptoms can get worse during times of stress. Depression also commonly occurs with the disorder, as it did in Martha's case, and is associated with worsening of symptoms. For most people, obsessive–compulsive disorder is diagnosed during late adolescence and early adulthood, but people typically report that some of their symptoms began to show during childhood. Although men may have an earlier age of onset, women are just slightly more likely to develop obsessive–compulsive disorder. The disorder is chronic if untreated.

To determine whether you might have obsessive–compulsive disorder, answer the following questions:

- Do you have recurring and unwanted ideas, thoughts, or impulses that you can't get out of your head despite your best efforts? These might include things such as thinking about harming a friend or relative, being overly concerned about germs and dirt, or fearing that you've forgotten to lock the door.
- Do you feel a need to perform certain actions repeatedly, finding them hard to resist? This might include things such as washing your hands repeatedly, checking over and over that you have locked the door or turned off the stove, counting before doing something, or thinking a "good" thought for every "bad" thought you have.

If you answered *yes* to either of these questions, there is a chance that you may have obsessive–compulsive disorder. If you like, you can conduct a more detailed self-test of your symptoms. You can do so easily by visiting the websites of the National Institute of Mental Health, the Obsessive–Compulsive Foundation, or the Anxiety Disorders Association of America and completing their online screening tests. Scoring procedures are provided on the websites. These tests, like other self-assessment tests described in this book, are usually used by doctors and researchers. They do have limitations. You can use them to help determine your specific symptoms and to discuss them with your doctor or mental health professional. As with panic disorder, treating obsessions and compulsions can often reduce health-related worries. So they're often the first targets for treatment. Some treatment options for obsessive–compulsive disorder are discussed at the end of this chapter.

Generalized Anxiety Disorder

Generalized anxiety disorder involves *excessive* and *uncontrollable* worry about everyday things that occurs more days than not for a period of at least six months. People with this disorder usually anticipate the worst possible outcome for whatever it is that they are worried about, although there usually aren't any signs of real trouble. They also find it very difficult not to worry. The focus of the worry can range from the important to the ordinary. For example, the worry may be about work-related or school-related matters, relationships, getting the bills paid, the health and well-being of oneself or loved ones, being late for an appointment, getting a chore done, and so on. Common symptoms include:

- Restlessness,
- Fatigue,
- Concentration difficulties,
- Irritability,
- Muscle tension, and
- Difficulties falling or staying asleep.

Because we all worry at times, it's difficult to identify a point at which normal worry becomes excessive. DSM-IV-TR suggests that this point occurs when the worry begins to cause a lot of distress or difficulties in important areas of day-to-day functioning.

Jenn: "I'm going to get kicked out of the graduate program."

Jenn, a 26-year-old graduate student, went to her doctor complaining that she was having difficulty falling and staying asleep. She was also having headaches almost every day that interfered with her ability to focus and concentrate. Jenn was currently worried about several things. First, she worried that her headaches might be related to the onset of some serious and life-threatening disease. She requested an MRI to see if this was the case. Second, because of her recent lack of sleep and poor concentration, she worried that her professor might not find her research to be of high enough quality. She reported frequently waking during the night and feeling very anxious about her many school-related responsibilities. "I worry that I'm going to get kicked out of the graduate program." She also reported being extremely irritable and tense. During the evaluation the doctor determined that Jenn's headaches were less frequent during a recent vacation and that she consistently received positive feedback from her professor. In fact, she had the best marks in her class. Her physical examination and lab tests all indicated her health to be good.

To be diagnosed with generalized anxiety disorder, you must have excessive anxiety and worry. This anxiety and worry must occur more days than not over a six-month period, must be about a number of events or activities, and can't be limited to anxiety and worry that's related to other mental health conditions. For example, your anxiety and worry can't just be about having another panic attack, as is the case in panic disorder. Nor can it just be about having a serious disease, as is the case in hypochondriasis. As we mentioned before, the anxiety and worry need to cause distress or impairment in day-to-day activities. As with the other anxiety disorders, a doctor needs to establish that the anxiety and worry aren't due to the effects of a drug or medication or a general medical condition such as hyperthyroidism or respiratory conditions. Jenn met all of these conditions and, as a result, was diagnosed with generalized anxiety disorder.

About 5 percent of the population will experience generalized anxiety disorder at some point during their lives. It can develop at any age but appears to be less prevalent in children than adults. In children and teens the focus of worry is often related to doing well in school and sports. Women are just slightly more likely than men to develop generalized anxiety disorder. Other conditions associated with stress—insomnia, headache, and irritable bowel syndrome—commonly happen at the same time as this disorder. So do depression and some of the other anxiety disorders.

Determining whether you might have generalized anxiety disorder involves figuring out (1) how often you worry, (2) how many things you worry about, and (3) how your worry influences your life. Take a moment to answer the following questions:

- Have you been worrying about things, more days than not, during the past six months?
- Do you worry about many different things despite there being no real signs of trouble? This might include worrying about failing a class despite having good grades or about not being able to pay the bills despite having a stable and well-paying job, worrying about your marriage despite having a great relationship with your spouse, and worrying that something terrible will happen to a loved one despite knowing that their health is good.
- Do you have a hard time controlling your worry?
- Does your worry cause you distress or interfere with your ability to function during the day?

If you answered *yes* to all of these questions, there's a strong possibility that you have generalized anxiety disorder. We recommend that you discuss these symptoms with your doctor or mental health professional. If you do have generalized anxiety disorder, it'll be easier to break the heath anxiety cycle *after* you get your general worry under control. And, as with panic and obsessive–compulsive disorders, treating generalized anxiety disorder often leads to a big reduction in health anxiety. Possible treatment options for generalized anxiety disorder are outlined in the last section of this chapter.

Helpful Hint

People with health anxiety often have another anxiety disorder at the same time. The anxiety disorders that have the most in common with health anxiety are panic disorder, obsessive–compulsive disorder, and generalized anxiety disorder. If the self-assessment exercises you did earlier indicate that you might have one or more of these disorders, we strongly recommend that you discuss your symptoms with your doctor or mental health professional. You can also discuss the various treatment options described later and determine whether one might be appropriate for you.

The Other Anxiety Disorders

We won't discuss other anxiety disorders—specific phobias, social phobia, post-traumatic stress disorder, acute stress disorder, anxiety disorder due to a general medical condition, or substance-induced anxiety disorder—in detail. A person may have any of these disorders along with health anxiety. But because they have less in common with health anxiety than panic disorder, obsessive–compulsive disorder, and generalized anxiety disorder, they're less likely to complicate health-related worries. If you feel that you might have one of these other anxiety disorders, you can refer to the listing of additional reading materials and related websites in the resource section at the end of this book.

Health Anxiety and the Overlapping Anxiety Disorders

Why do some of the anxiety disorders share characteristics with health anxiety? Some researchers believe it's because they have similar causes. These causes might be biological in nature. They might also be related to the ways in which people pay attention to and interpret things that they experience (as we discussed in Chapter 2). Most likely it's some combination of these possibilities. At this point we really don't know. What we do know, however, is that all forms of anxiety produce sensations in the body and that people with health anxiety believe that these sensations mean that they are physically ill.

It's important to know whether you also have one of the anxiety disorders discussed here, because, if you do, it will be more difficult for you to manage your health anxiety. This is especially true for panic disorder because the symptoms often cause bodily sensations, such as a rapidly pounding heart, that can be perceived as being dangerous to your health. It's also true in cases of obsessive–compulsive disorder and generalized anxiety disorder, such as those of Martha and Jenn presented earlier, in which you may be concerned about catching or having a serious disease. We can't overstate the importance of your looking into these conditions if you suspect you have one of them. Sometimes learning to cope with these anxiety disorders can be the most effective way of reducing your health-related worries.

Treatment Options for Anxiety Disorders

People with one of the anxiety disorders described here have a number of treatment options. Choosing a particular method of treatment is often a matter of preference. Some people prefer taking medications, whereas others opt for one of the various forms of psychotherapy. Here we briefly describe some of the more popular options (and ones for which there is evidence of effectiveness).

Medication

Several medications are effective in reducing the anxiety associated with panic disorder, obsessive–compulsive disorder, and generalized anxiety disorder. For panic disorder these include medications such as the *selective serotonin reuptake inhibitor* (SSRI) antidepressant medications Paxil, Zoloft, Serzone, and Celexa. The benzodiazepine medications Xanax, Ativan, and Klonopin also work well for people who panic (but their effects may not last as long as those of the SSRI antidepressants). Obsessive–compulsive disorder is often effectively treated with Anafranil and the SSRI medications Prozac, Luvox, Paxil, and Zoloft. Buspar and the SSRI medications Paxil, Zoloft, Luvox, and Serzone are effective in relieving symptoms of generalized anxiety disorder. Common side effects for these SSRIs are shown in Table 4 in Chapter 4.

Advantages of medications are that they're usually covered by health insurance and that they are available to almost everybody who can get to a doctor. Cost and where one lives aren't obstacles to this treatment option. A disadvantage is that medications work only if your doctor has prescribed the right medication for you and your symptoms and only if you take them as directed by your doctor. Possible side effects can occur that you should consider. Discuss these side effects with your doctor and ask for information pamphlets on the medications you consider taking. In Chapter 10, we discuss medication options for treating health anxiety.

Cognitive-Behavioral Therapy

Cognitive-behavioral therapy is a form of treatment offered primarily by mental health professionals—psychiatrists and psychologists. It involves a number of different strategies, including psychoeducation, cognitive restructuring, relaxation exercises, and various forms of exposure and response prevention.

- *Psychoeducation* involves giving people information about a particular disorder so that they can understand it better.
- *Cognitive restructuring* focuses on getting people to rethink mistaken beliefs that they hold and to replace these with alternative (and more realistic) ways of thinking about their concerns.
- Relaxation and anxiety are opposing responses that do not occur together. Therefore, *relaxation exercises* designed to reduce muscle tension and promote deep breathing are taught as a way to reduce the effects of anxiety. These exercises can be used as part of a therapy program or, as described later, on their own as a general way of coping with stress.
- *Exposure and response prevention* is a combined strategy that involves exposing people to situations that worsen their anxiety and then preventing them from doing the behaviors that they perform as a way of dealing with their anxiety. This teaches the person that these behaviors are unnecessary. Exposure to bodily sensations can also be used alone when the goal of the therapist is to show that the sensations are harmless.

The specific focus of these strategies depends on the anxiety disorder being treated. For example, in treating panic disorder, the therapist might use an exposure exercise such as running up a flight of stairs to demonstrate that a pounding heart does not necessarily signal a heart attack. In treating obsessive–compulsive disorder, the therapist would most likely combine exposure to situations that aggravate obsessions, such as having Martha change a dirty diaper, with preventing her from washing her child's rear and her hands more than once.

An advantage of cognitive-behavioral therapy is that it teaches ways of dealing with anxiety—usually over a period of 12 weeks or so—that have lasting effects and that can be used again in the future if anxiety resurfaces. Disadvantages are that it's not covered by all health plans and that it requires access over a long period of time to a trained therapist. This can be difficult for people who don't live in a large urban area and have to travel to see the therapist. In Chapter 10 we describe how cognitive-behavioral therapy is used to treat health anxiety.

Other Forms of Psychotherapy

Other forms of psychotherapy, including hypnosis and approaches based more on the teachings and style of Sigmund Freud, have been used in the treatment of the anxiety disorders. The research provides little support for the effectiveness of these approaches. For this reason we don't discuss them further. Nor do we recommend them.

Self-Help

Many self-help treatments are available for anxiety disorders. These range from learning how to relax and learning ways to manage stress to exercising and eating properly. Step-by-step programs designed for each of the anxiety disorders are also available. Self-help strategies provide the distinct advantage of not requiring direct involvement from a physician or mental health professional, and, in many cases, they cost very little. They also allow you to assume responsibility for managing your road to recovery. A disadvantage is that they require considerable (and often unassisted) effort on your part. You can get further information on self-help programs for many of the anxiety disorders by referring to the Resources section at the end of this book. Strategies to assist you in dealing with your health anxiety are described in detail in Parts II and III of this book.

Combined and Sequential Treatments

Is there a benefit to combining treatments or to receiving them one after the other? There's little evidence to suggest that combining treatments for an anxiety disorder is a more effective strategy than receiving one treatment alone. Many people are able to effectively manage their anxiety using self-help, cognitive-behavioral therapy, or medication alone. When one treatment is giving you good results, it would seem wasteful to add another. If, however, you find that you hit a roadblock with a particular treatment, then you might consider adding another. This is referred to as a sequential approach. For example, you might start by trying a self-help program but, after having some success, realize that help from a therapist or medication may be needed to make further gains. Or, if your symptoms are severe, you might want to begin with medication for fast relief and gradually taper off while doing a self-help or therapy program.

Things to Remember

Several of the anxiety disorders can occur at the same time as health anxiety. You need to know whether you have one of these other anxiety disorders—particularly panic disorder, obsessive–compulsive disorder, or generalized anxiety disorder—because they can make it more difficult for you to get your health anxiety under control. Use the questions that we provided to determine whether you have symptoms of one of these anxiety disorders. If so, discuss these symptoms further with your doctor or a mental health professional. Also, with the understanding that treatment can come in several different forms, you can discuss treatment options and determine which is right for you. In some cases, getting treatment for an anxiety disorder that overlaps with health anxiety will greatly reduce your health-related worries.

Four

Sick and Sad
Am I Depressed, Too?

Sadness and depression often occur at the same time as health anxiety problems. This makes perfect sense: When you worry a lot about something, you tend not to feel particularly cheerful. Worrying takes a lot of energy and can be tiring. It can affect your ability to sleep. It can consume your attention to the point at which you have little interest in anything else. And it can make you irritable and cranky. Also people who are depressed frequently become preoccupied with the functioning of their bodies and worry about having a serious disease. These things add up to create an overall miserable state. They also, unfortunately, complicate a person's life by increasing unwanted somatic sensations and taxing already limited coping resources. The degree of complication depends directly on how depressed a person feels and whether the depression started before or after the health anxiety.

In this chapter we'll introduce you to the types of depression commonly experienced by people with health anxiety—major depressive disorder and dysthymic disorder—and provide you with some tools that will allow you to determine how depressed you are. We'll also explain the primary reasons depression and health anxiety can occur at the same time. Why is this important? Depression can reduce the likelihood that you'll be successful in overcoming your health-related worries. So our goal in this chapter is to help you determine whether you should be seeking help for depression before you begin our program for taking control of your health worries.

Common Mood Disorders

Marilyn: "I have no interest in anything."

Marilyn is a 38-year-old woman who has been married for 15 years and has two school-age children. Since her teenage years she's experienced recurring episodes of depression, lasting five or six months at a time. Individual and family psychotherapy, along with antidepressant medication, has reduced her depression in the past. Although she was free from depression for three years, her symptoms returned with a vengeance about four months ago. At first she was feeling irritable and cranky, but within a week or two she became discouraged about anything and everything. She now describes herself as feeling "sad, tearful, and completely worthless" and reports having lost interest in pretty much everything she once enjoyed. She feels this way most of the time and can't think of more than one occasion in the past few months when she's laughed or smiled. Marilyn hasn't been at work for the past six weeks and prior to that had been calling in sick a lot. She simply has no energy and wants to do nothing but sleep. Since being at home, she's been unable to enjoy spending time with her kids and, in fact, has noticed a growing lack of interest in being around them at all. "They bug me. They get on my nerves. I just want them to leave me alone and stop waking me up." She finds this very disheartening, and it makes her feel very guilty. So does her growing lack of interest in her husband. "We were getting along great until this started again. Now I don't want to listen to what he's got to say. I don't want to be around him. And I've got absolutely no interest in making love. I'm sure he thinks I'm a good-for-nothing lazy blob anyway." In the past few weeks she's become concerned about the possible causes of aches and pains in her joints and muscles and this, combined with her growing feelings of guilt, prompted her to think about visiting her doctor.

Depression is a word that our society uses to refer to feelings of intense sadness or despair. *Major depressive disorder* is the name used by the American Psychiatric Association in DSM-IV-TR to describe a common form of depression. The differences between Marilyn's depression and the feelings of sadness or unhappiness that we all experience from time to time are the severity and duration of symptoms. Major depression is characterized by a deep sense of sadness or a lack of interest in or enjoyment of just about everything. Some people experience both deep sadness and lack of interest or enjoyment. Several other symptoms might also be present. These include:

- Increases or decreases in weight (when not dieting),
- Changes in appetite,
- Too much or too little sleep,
- Restlessness,
- Lack of energy,
- Feelings of worthlessness, shame, or guilt,
- Inability to concentrate or make decisions, and
- Thoughts of dying or committing suicide.

If these symptoms occur most of the day, nearly every day over a two-week period or longer, major depression may be diagnosed. This was the case for Marilyn. The symptoms also have to represent a change from the way the person was previously (Marilyn had been happy and active for three years prior to the return of her depression), they have to cause distress or affect home and work activities (Marilyn had withdrawn from her family and had stopped working), and they can't simply be part of grieving after the loss of a loved one. The severity of major depression, although greater than temporary states of day-to-day sadness, can itself range from mild to severe. People with more severe cases of major depression usually have greater difficulty functioning at home and work and are likely to be suicidal. Adults who are depressed tend to pay a lot of attention to their bodies and worry a lot that bodily sensations may be signals for disease.

Major depression is fairly common. About 3 percent of men and up to 9 percent of women meet the criteria for diagnosis of a current episode of major depression. That means that 1 in every 20 people have major depression right now! And anywhere from 5 to 12 percent of men and 10 to 25 percent of women will experience major depression at some point during their lifetimes. Depression can begin in childhood, adolescence, or adulthood, and it tends to be recurring (that is, it comes and goes). Symptoms worsen over a period of days to weeks before reaching the level that warrants a diagnosis of major depression. In most cases, if left untreated, they last for months. Most people with major depression experience full or partial remission of symptoms (particularly when treated) but, for an unfortunate few, the symptoms can last for years without relief.

Dysthymic disorder, or dysthymia, is another common form of depression. It occurs in about 6 percent of the population at some point during their lives. Dysthymia involves feelings of sadness that last most of the day for nearly every day over a period of two years or more. People with this type of depression usually report that they're "down in the dumps" and that they've felt this way for as long as they can remember. Dysthymia is diagnosed when:

- The person has a depressed mood and several other symptoms (such as changes in appetite or sleep patterns, low self-esteem) lasting longer than two years,
- The symptoms don't qualify for a diagnosis of major depression, and
- He or she hasn't had a symptom-free period for more than two months at a time.

There are subtle yet important differences between dysthymia and major depression. First, symptoms of dysthymia are moderate in severity but can be so long lasting that they're seen as a usual part of the person; he or she has always been that way. Major depression, on the other hand, involves episodes of severe changes in mood that are unlike the way the person usually acts. Second, people with dysthymia have fewer changes in their sleep patterns, appetite, or weight and less restlessness than do those with major depression. The two conditions are otherwise quite similar. Not surprisingly, dysthymia is a risk factor for major depression. That is, if you have it you're more likely to develop major depression than if you don't have it.

You can ask yourself several questions to help decide whether you have one of these types of clinical depression.

- Do you feel cranky, sad, or "down in the dumps"?
- Have you lost interest or been displeased in the things you once enjoyed?
- Has your weight increased or decreased a lot?
- Have you noticed changes in your sleep patterns, for example, sleeping much more or much less than usual?
- Have you been restless?
- Do you feel tired or as though you don't have any energy?
- Do you feel worthless, ashamed, or guilty about things?
- Have you had trouble concentrating or making decisions?
- Do you feel hopeless?
- Have you though a lot about death or about killing yourself?
- Have you tried to take your own life?

If you answered *yes* to *at least one of the first two questions*, as well as four of the others, there is a pretty good possibility that you have major depression. If you've been feeling sad or "down" for most of the past two years or more but have only a couple of other symptoms, you may have dysthymia. If you think you may be depressed, we want you to have your symptoms checked out professionally. Remember, just like the anxiety disorders discussed in Chapter 3, only an evaluation by a doctor or mental health professional can determine whether you actually have one of these disorders. And, if you do, helpful treatments are available.

Links between Health Anxiety and Depression

Whether you have one of the more severe and long-lasting types of depression or are just feeling a little "down in the dumps," understanding the relationship between depression and health anxiety is an important step in taking back control of your life. Let's have a closer look at how they're related and what you can do to renew your zest for living.

Our experience has consistently shown us that health anxiety and depression are closely linked—many of our patients have both. There are several explanations for this. Some researchers believe health-related worries are always a by-product of other conditions, including some of the anxiety disorders discussed in Chapter 3, but especially depression. They argue that depressed people become concerned with bodily sensations and that, as a result of their negative outlook on life, they become preoccupied with the idea that they are physically ill. Think about some of the symptoms of depression. Poor sleep, changes in routine and diet, inactivity. What do these things do? As we pointed out in Chapter 2, they all cause unwanted noise in the body. ("I'm feeling a lot of pain in my stomach and bowels. Maybe I have some sort of gastric problem. An ulcer? Maybe it's something worse, like cancer.") Other symptoms of depression, such as sluggishness or inability to concentrate, can also be misinterpreted as symptoms of disease. "Wow, am I ever short on energy. Clumsy too! I really hope it's not multiple sclerosis." Coupling these sorts of beliefs with feelings of sadness and despair—that nothing's right in the world—makes it more likely that you'll believe that something's seriously wrong with your body.

Other researchers suggest that constantly worrying about your health and well-being can lead to negative changes in mood; that is, the process of worrying about your health, checking for signs of worsening, and seeking reassurance that everything is okay (despite not really believing it is) can leave you feeling that life is hopeless. This seems logical. It's discouraging when doctors repeatedly tell you that there's nothing physically wrong with you when you believe something *is* wrong. It's disheartening to think that you're sick and dying from some disease that nobody seems to have any interesting in finding or helping you overcome. It's difficult to realize you should be spending time with your loved ones when you really have no interest in anything but finding out what's going on in your body. In some people the feelings of despair and hopelessness that result from constant worry can actually persist or worsen to the point at which a diagnosis of dysthymia or major depression is warranted.

We believe both of these explanations are correct: Some people are depressed first and then develop health anxiety about depression-related bodily sensations, whereas others have health-related worries that later affect their mood. Determining which group you fit into has important implications for the path we recommend you take to overcoming your health worries. Here's what we recommend:

- If your mood changes developed *after* you began worrying a lot about your health, then you can proceed with the strategies outlined in the remainder of this book. They will help you take back control of your life.
- If your depression was present *before* your health anxiety, then the path to recovery is a little different. We, like many therapists, believe that if depression came first, then it's the first issue that needs to be tackled and

overcome. Some of the treatment options you should consider are outlined next. Treating your depression may completely alleviate your health anxiety, particularly if your concerns are about bodily sensations that are directly related to depression. Or it might provide partial relief, in which case you can return to the book and start using our strategies to overcome your remaining health worries.

Treatment Options for Depression

Many treatment options are available for people who have major depression or dysthymia. People with severe cases of depression, especially those who are suicidal or have recently attempted suicide, may need to be hospitalized. For most others, the options include one of various types of antidepressant medications, as well as several forms of psychotherapy. Medication and psychotherapy are often combined. As with the anxiety disorders, picking a particular method of treatment is a matter of personal preference. In the following sections, we've provided a brief summary of some of the more popular options (and, in keeping with the scientists within us, ones that have proven evidence of effectiveness).

Medication

Medication is the most common treatment for depression. It's often started with a visit to the family doctor. Your doctor may ask such questions as "Have you been feeling sad and depressed? For how long? Have you been sleeping more than usual?" in order to determine whether or not to prescribe an antidepressant medication. Unfortunately, many people who are prescribed antidepressants by their family doctors don't get the medication for long enough periods of time or in adequate doses for it to be effective. The result is that a potentially helpful medication may have little effect on depression because the prescription runs out before it's had a chance to work. It can take five or six weeks to find out whether an antidepressant is working properly and without unpleasant side effects. After that, it can take several more months for the medication to have its full effect on your symptoms.

Some family doctors have a habit of paying little attention to the impact of depression on your ability to get along well and function in day-to-day living at home and work. This is understandable: They see many patients each day who have many different kinds of health problems, and they can't be expected to have expert knowledge of each one. Because of this, we think it's a good idea to ask your doctor for a referral to a psychiatrist so that all aspects of your depression are considered in planning your treatment. In addition to providing a complete assessment of your condition, the psychiatrist has a more thorough knowledge about antidepressant medications and how they work.

They're also trained to recognize when psychotherapy may be beneficial, and they can prescribe and provide a treatment approach that combines medication and psychotherapy.

Antidepressant medications come in several varieties. They all work a little differently on the chemical systems in the body that are thought to be involved in depression. The monoamine oxidase inhibitors (MAOIs) such as Marplan, Manerix, and Parnate, have been available for over half a century. As their name suggests, they reduce levels of monoamine oxidase—a protein in the brain responsible for cleaning up other brain chemicals—and thereby allow other brain chemicals that make us feel good, such as norepinephrine and serotonin, to be active. Tricyclic antidepressants, such as Elavil and Tofranil, have also been around for many years. But because they cause considerable drowsiness and can have other serious or unwanted side effects, they aren't typically the first choice for many. Newer tricyclic antidepressants, such as Norpramin and Pamelor, seem to have fewer effects on alertness and thus are more common choices. Some newer medicines, such as Wellbutrin (a tricyclic that has a stimulating rather than a sedating effect) and Effexor (a drug that prevents the body from reabsorbing norepinephrine and serotonin), have become commonly used in recent years. The SSRIs have been and remain the most commonly prescribed antidepressants over the past 10 years. They appear to be less likely to cause drowsiness and to have fewer serious side effects than do many of the other antidepressants. The SSRIs, especially Prozac, have been shown to be effective in reducing health anxiety. Table 4 shows the SSRIs approved for use in the United States, as well as their common side effects.

The advantages and disadvantages of taking medication to control depression are the same as those for anxiety—they're usually covered by insurance, but they work only if the right one is prescribed (for the right amount of time) and if they're taken as directed by your doctor or psychiatrist. Your doctor or psychiatrist may base his or her decision of which medication is best for you, in part, on the following:

- Whether a particular antidepressant has worked for you or a close relative in the past,
- The specific symptoms you are experiencing, and
- Your physical health and lifestyle.

You need to be sure that your doctor or psychiatrist understands the extent of your health anxiety. This may affect the medication you're prescribed. Remember that Prozac and some of the other SSRIs can reduce symptoms of both depression and health anxiety. If your doctor seems to be unaware of this, don't be afraid to take an active role in planning your treatment by having a discussion with him or her about whether an SSRI is the best medication option for you.

TABLE 4. Profiles of Selective Serotonin Reuptake Inhibitors Approved in the United States for Treating Depression

Common name	Typical dose (milligrams)	Most common side effects	
Celexa	20–50	• Anxiety • Sleepiness • Nausea	• Headache • Trouble sleeping
Luvox	150–400	• Sleepiness • Trouble sleeping • Anxiety • Tremor • Nausea	• Loss of appetite • Vomiting • Sweating • Delayed orgasm • Diarrhea
Paxil	20–50	• Nausea • Sleepiness • Fatigue • Dizziness • Trouble sleeping	• Sweating • Tremor • Loss of appetite • Anxiety • Delayed orgasm
Prozac	20–100	• Agitation • Anxiety • Trouble sleeping • Sleepiness • Tremor • Loss of appetite	• Nausea • Diarrhea • Headache • Dizziness • Delayed orgasm
Zoloft	50–300	• Nausea • Diarrhea • Tremor • Dizziness • Trouble sleeping	• Sleepiness • Sweating • Dry mouth • Delayed orgasm

Cognitive-Behavioral Therapy

Cognitive-behavioral therapy is another effective way of treating symptoms of depression. It can be at least as effective as medication for current symptoms. Also, the skills learned in therapy are very helpful in reducing the chances of depression returning with full force again in the future (as happened with Marilyn). This is an important thing to consider when selecting a treatment, because most people who are depressed now will experience a return of their symptoms to some degree at some time in the future.

Treating depression with cognitive-behavioral therapy usually takes about five or six months. Although treatment can be set up in many different ways, a typical treatment plan would involve 15 to 25 one-hour sessions that are attended once weekly. Booster sessions can be scheduled as needed so that important skills aren't forgotten.

This treatment works by changing the cognitive distortions—or what we call *negative ways of thinking*—that go hand in hand with depression. People with depression can have cognitive distortions about many different things in their lives, including the way they think about themselves ("I'm worthless."), their world as a whole ("I can't handle all of the demands people are making. Work. The kids. Keeping the house in order. Augh!"), and their future ("Things are hopeless. Nothing I do seems to make a difference.")

Marilyn had many of these kinds of thoughts. She was feeling so worthless that she eventually started thinking that everybody disliked her. "I've pushed my kids away. My best friend hasn't called or stopped by lately. Oh well, it doesn't really matter anyway." A cognitive-behavioral therapist would work with Marilyn to come up with other explanations for her beliefs about why her husband, kids, and friends weren't around as much lately. Perhaps her friend has been very busy with other things or even away during the past few weeks. Her family may be trying to respect her wishes to be left alone. Marilyn's therapist used psychoeducation and cognitive restructuring (techniques we described in Chapter 3) to help her change her negative way of thinking about things. She also had Marilyn stick to a regular schedule of activities that she had once enjoyed (for example, spending 20 minutes each evening doing puzzles with her kids and going to the gym for a light workout every second day).

When depressed people change distortions and inaccuracies in their thinking about themselves, the world around them, and their future, positive changes occur in their moods and their behavior. They regain a more positive outlook on life and begin enjoying the things they liked to do before becoming depressed.

Other Forms of Psychotherapy

Interpersonal therapy focuses on the role that relationships play in depression. The idea is that all depressed people have difficulties in their relationships with other people and that these difficulties make depression worse. Fixing the interpersonal trouble spots should, therefore, reduce the severity of depression. Grief about the end of an important relationship, a new role at home or work, ongoing conflicts with another person, and shortcomings in social or communication skills are usually the focus of this type of therapy. A typical treatment plan might consist of weekly sessions that last for about 16 weeks in total. As with cognitive-behavioral therapy, booster sessions can be scheduled as needed. Research has shown that interpersonal therapy is effective in reducing depression. It has been shown to work as well as medication and cognitive-behavioral therapy.

A variety of other psychotherapies—for example, marital and family therapy, as well as brief dynamic psychotherapy (an approach based on the teachings of Sigmund Freud)—have also been used to treat depression. The idea behind marital and family therapy is that unhealthy family relationships go hand in hand with depression. This sounds similar to interpersonal therapy, but marital and family therapy isn't specifically targeted at reducing symptoms of depression. It can be helpful in cases in which strained family relationships are contributing to a person's depression. Unfortunately, not enough research has been done to compare it against medication or more proven forms of psychotherapy. Psychodynamic psychotherapy was not designed specifically for treating depression, either. Like marital and family therapy, it hasn't been compared against other proven forms of depression treatment.

Combined Treatments

A few weeks after Marilyn had visited her doctor about her increasing depression, a psychiatrist evaluated her. The psychiatrist discussed possible treatment options with her. It was decided that a combination of antidepressants and cognitive-behavioral therapy would be best for her. The psychiatrist explained that this approach had the benefits of both worlds: The antidepressants have a more immediate impact on symptoms, and the cognitive-behavioral therapy provides a skill set that can be used to modify negative thinking and thereby reduce the chances of relapse. Some research supports this approach to treatment, suggesting that the amount of change in symptoms is greater when these treatment approaches are combined. People who receive a combination of antidepressants and cognitive-behavioral therapy or interpersonal therapy may have longer depression-free periods than those who receive only one type of treatment.

If your depression is severe and you want the more immediate relief of symptoms that antidepressants can bring, then starting with medication and following with one of the psychotherapies may be the best option for you. Again, don't be afraid to discuss this possibility with the person responsible for planning your treatment.

Things to Remember

Many people have depression. For some people it's severe enough to get in the way of their enjoying life and being able to do the things we all need to do to get by at home and work. Both minor sadness and more severe forms of depression can happen at the same time as health anxiety. Because major depression and dysthymia can get in the way of your taking control of your health anxiety, it's important for you to know whether you have one of these types of depression and to deal with it. If you think you have major depression or dysthymia, ask your doctor about your symptoms and some of the treatment options outlined here. Be sure your doctor understands the nature of your health anxiety (we discuss how to talk with your doctor about health anxiety in more detail in Chapter 8). We recommend that you ask your doctor for a referral to a psychiatrist or other mental health professional to get a more thorough assessment and specialized treatment planning. With the right treatment plan, you'll be able to conquer your depression while also reducing your health anxiety. Once your depression is under control, come back to the remaining chapters of this book. They'll give you the skills needed to further reduce your health anxiety, to keep it in check, and to stop it from interfering with your enjoyment of life.

Part II

BREAKING THE HEALTH ANXIETY CYCLE

Five

Understanding and Managing Stress

By now you have a pretty good idea about how much health anxiety you have. You also have a basic understanding of where your bodily sensations come from, how they can be misinterpreted as signs and symptoms of disease, and how the vicious cycle of health anxiety feeds itself. This is an excellent start. Over the years a large number of patients have told us that having a better understanding of what's going on in their bodies, combined with knowing that many other people are going through the same thing, has helped them break the anxiety cycle. This is precisely why cognitive-behavioral therapists include psychoeducation in their treatment programs. In this chapter we're going to move beyond teaching you about health anxiety and help you lay the foundation to start using our strategies to get your health anxiety under control.

As we mentioned in Chapter 1, you'll need to let yourself at least consider the *possibility* that the bodily sensations that cause you concern aren't disease related but instead are happening because of such things as stress and fatigue. We understand that you may still be skeptical about viewing your bodily sensations as part of anything other than disease. In Chapter 2 we asked you to rate how much you believe it's possible that your symptoms are the result of being stuck in the health anxiety cycle. Your rating may not have changed much yet, but if it's 1 or higher, we're still set to move forward. You've probably spent a lot of time consulting doctors, trying to figure out whether you have a serious disease. Don't you owe it to yourself to check out all the possible causes of your bodily concerns, such as stress and fatigue?

The key to better health might be in changing your ways of thinking and behaving rather than pinpointing a specific disease. It's okay if you're still a little uncomfortable with this idea. It's a change in the way you've been thinking about these things and in the way you've understood the functioning of your body. But it's a very important step. Are you willing to try giving up relying on others, such as doctors, to improve your health? Are you willing to take personal control of your situation? The fact that you're still reading this book is a good sign that you've already decided to think about doing this. Now, on a scale of 1 to 10, with 10 being the highest, rate how motivated or interested you are in trying out some of our strategies to help you overcome your health concerns. Ideally, we'd like your rating to be between 8 and 10. But, as before, if your rating was anything other than 0, we're ready to get started. Perhaps your motivation for trying our strategies will increase as we build on the information we've presented you with so far by showing you how to reduce your feelings of anxiety.

Your next step is to learn some basic skills for managing and coping with stress. We live in a world that can be hectic at the best of times. Stress is a fact of life. Stress management skills are tools that can come in handy when faced with stressful and difficult life circumstances. Also, we want you to have some basic strategies that can be used whenever you feel your health anxiety coming on or getting to a point that isn't manageable. Finally, to be frank, some of the exercises we'll have you practice in Chapters 6 and 7 will create thoughts and bodily sensations that will make you feel a little anxious. It may seem strange that we're going to make you anxious in order to help you with your anxiety, but there's a good reason for doing this: To triumph over anxiety, we need to confront the things that make us anxious. For example, people who are afraid of flying in airplanes eventually have to fly in an airplane to overcome their fear. This is a necessary part of breaking any anxiety cycle, including the health anxiety cycle.

By the end of this chapter you'll be prepared to counteract any anxiety you feel by relaxing your mind and body. You'll also be able to organize your life in a less stressful way. To accomplish these things, we're going to teach you several stress management strategies. The steps you'll work through look like this:

1. Identifying your stressors.
2. Understanding the stress reaction.
3. Learning relaxation strategies.
4. Learning how to breathe for relaxation.
5. Learning how to be an effective problem solver.
6. Learning good time management.

Identifying and Understanding the Things That Stress You Out

On a typical weekday, most people spend 10 or 11 hours working and getting to and from work, 4 hours doing various household chores and child-care activities, and 7 or 8 hours sleeping. That's about 22 hours of the day! Not much time for anything else, let alone personal interests and leisure. It's no wonder that stress is something everyone experiences on a day-to-day basis. We believe strongly that the ability to successfully manage stress is a skill that forms the foundation of any program that aims to reduce anxiety. Our primary objective for this chapter is to have you learn how to be a good manager of your own stress.

People tend to think of stress as something in their surroundings. We often hear someone say that they're stressed out by the demands of work, not having enough time in the day to get things done, or not having enough money to pay the bills. The sources of stress are often referred to as *stressors*. Other common stressors include strained relationships, illnesses in the family, child rearing, legal problems, and things that seem to needlessly use up time (such as waiting in slow-moving lines or being stuck in traffic). Add to this the burden of constant worry about health, and the day-to-day begins to look almost insurmountable! Take a minute to identify the stressors you've experienced over the past week by completing Worksheet 2. We'd be surprised if there weren't at least three or four circles on your worksheet. The good news is that you can learn to manage your stress and the things that cause it.

Rather than viewing stress as something that happens outside of a person (in his or her surroundings), we like to think of it as a process of dealing with those things that place demands on a person and his or her time and abilities. When the demands placed on a person exceed his or her resources for dealing with the demands, stress reactions occur. *Stress reactions* include emotional distress, such as feeling all wound up or overwhelmed, as well as some combination of one or more of the harmless but uncomfortable bodily sensations listed in Worksheet 3.

It might not be obvious, but there are links between your stressors and at least some of the bodily sensations you experience. To determine which bodily sensations are stress related, try the following. Keep a diary of stressors that occur during each day over the next week. Record the bodily sensations that accompany your response to each stressor you identify. When you examine the diary at the end of the week, you'll find that you characteristically experience certain bodily sensations as part of your stress reaction. For example, when Joan (see Chapter 1) worked through this exercise, she was surprised to find how consistently her nausea and stomach upset occurred during the times she was running late and unable to keep up with things.

Because the stress reaction includes harmless bodily sensations that you misinterpret as signs or symptoms of disease, strategies that reduce the stress reaction can also reduce health anxiety. How does this work? These strategies teach you to:

- Recognize bodily sensations as a harmless part of the stress reaction rather than as signs or symptoms of disease, and
- Reduce the strength of your stress reaction and how often it occurs.

Worksheet 2. Common Stressors

Stress is a fact of life, although people commonly fail to recognize how it affects them. This is because stressors are often minor irritants or hassles. When hassles do occur, people often experience stress-related bodily sensations. This is especially likely when many stressors occur at the same time or in succession. The following are some common stressors. Circle the ones that you experienced in the past week.

Household

Difficulty arranging child care
Too many household chores
Shopping problems
Crowded living space
Difficulties with home maintenance
Misplacing or losing things
Conflicts with partner or children
Divorce or separation
Car trouble

Social

Too few friends
Feeling isolated
Friends or relatives living too far away
Arguments with friends
Dating problems
Unwanted social obligations

Neighborhood and environment

Weather (for example, too hot, too cold, too humid)
Things that you are allergic to
Pollution
Crime
Traffic
Commuting
Noise
Waiting lines
Neighborhood crowding
Troublesome neighbors
Inconsiderate smokers
Parking problems
Problems with other drivers
Discrimination or harassment
Disturbing news stories

Work

Difficult duties
Inadequate training
Lack of a clear job description
Lack of appreciation
No avenue to voice concerns
Insufficient resources
Boring job
Doing job below level of competence
Concerns about shift work
Insufficient backup
Long work hours
A lot of responsibility with little or no authority
Unrealistic deadlines or expectations
Conflict with coworkers
Incompetent colleagues
Hassles from boss
Problems with supervisees
Staff shortages
Difficult clients
Computer problems (hardware or software)
Difficulty keeping up with technological developments
Poor promotional prospects
Unpleasant working conditions (for example, noisy, dirty, no privacy, cramped)
Too much travel (for example, to meetings)
Lack of work boundaries (that is, being contacted after hours by e-mail, phone, or pager)
Corporate downsizing, restructuring, or job relocation
Workplace violence
Lack of job security
Unemployment

(cont.)

School or university

Conflicts with roommates
Conflicts with other students or instructors
Academic deadlines
Difficult or boring courses
Too much schoolwork
Concerns about career path
Financial problems (for example, problems
  with student loans)
Budgeting problems

Finances

Debts
Credit problems
Lack of money to pay bills
Insufficient money for recreational activities
  (for example, movies)
Problems with taxes
Retirement concerns
Auto payments

Time pressures

Too much to do
Too little to do
Too many interruptions
Insufficient time for recreation
Too many meetings
Too many responsibilities

Health

Physical illness
Physical disability
Concerns with medical treatment
Treatment side effects
Concerns about physical appearance
Overweight
Underweight
Sexual problems

Inner concerns

Inability to express oneself
Conflicts about life choices (for example,
  career, choice of dating partner)
Too much time on one's hands
Concerns about the meaning of life
Too little sleep

Legal

Parking tickets
Speeding fines
Other legal problems

Other stressors in your life (please list)

ILLNESS OF FAMILY MEMBER

Source: From S. Taylor and G. J. G. Asmundson (2004). *Treating health anxiety: A cognitive-behavioral approach*. New York: Guilford Press. Reprinted by permission.

Worksheet 3. Common Stress-Related Bodily Reactions

Stressors, big and small, can produce bodily reactions. Sometimes these reactions happen while you are experiencing a stressful event, and sometimes they occur later on. The following is a list of some of the common stress-related bodily reactions. Not all of these sensations occur together; people typically experience one or two (or sometimes more) of these sensations during times of stress. Circle the ones that you have experienced in the past week. For each bodily sensation you circled, rate how much it bothered you over the past week by placing a number from 1 (*not very bothersome*) to 10 (*extremely bothersome*) on the line beside the sensation.

_____ Muscle spasms   _____ Stomach cramps

_____ Chest pain   _____ Nausea

_____ Feeling restless or fidgety   _____ Indigestion

_____ Fatigue   _____ Stomach churning

_____ Headache   _____ Diarrhea

_____ Neck pain   _____ Frequent need to urinate

_____ Chest tightness   _____ Difficulty swallowing

_____ Leg cramps   _____ Weight gain

_____ Backache   _____ Weight loss

_____ Aches and pains   _____ Heart thumping

_____ Trembling   _____ Heart racing

_____ Difficulty taking a deep breath   _____ Heart skipping a beat

_____ Tingling in the feet or hands   _____ Dry mouth

_____ Muscle twitches   _____ Dizziness

_____ Hot flashes   _____ Feeling light-headed

_____ Sweating   _____ Insomnia

Source: Adapted from S. Taylor and G. J. G. Asmundson (2004). *Treating health anxiety: A cognitive-behavioral approach*. New York: Guilford Press. Adapted by permission.

Our approach to stress management involves several strategies that promote relaxation (applied relaxation training and breathing retraining), as well as training in problem solving and time management, in order to better equip you to deal with workload demands and other time pressures related to living your life. Because each of the exercises presented in this chapter can have positive influences on your success with the other exercises, we strongly recommend that you practice and become proficient with each one in the order presented before moving on to the next one.

Learning to Relax: Weeks 1 to 3

Applied relaxation is more than kicking back and unwinding after a busy day. It's a series of exercises that were originally designed by Swedish psychologist Lars Goran Öst to counteract the stress reaction. Öst and others have shown that applied relaxation can:

- Stop the build-up of substances released by the body as part of the stress reaction, allowing your body to recover from the potentially damaging effects they can have on your cardiovascular system;
- Prevent the troubling (but harmless) bodily sensations, such as those listed in Worksheet 3, that are part of the stress reaction;
- Help you let go of your worries;
- Increase your energy level;
- Increase your ability to focus on tasks;
- Improve the soundness of your sleep; and
- Increase your self-confidence and feelings of personal control.

The basic principle on which applied relaxation is based is that our bodies aren't capable of being both stressed (a sympathetic nervous system "fight-or-flight" response) and relaxed (a parasympathetic nervous system "business as usual" response) at the same time. Learning to relax on demand will, therefore, reduce your stress and associated bodily sensations. Although it will take a couple of weeks of consistent practice to master our applied relaxation technique, you will become much better able to get through a stressful day and actually kick back for a bit at its conclusion. The payoff is worth the effort!

Our approach to applied relaxation involves three exercises. Each one takes about one week to become proficient at. The exercises are called tense–release relaxation (week 1), release-only relaxation (week 2), and rapid relaxation (week 3). With practice you'll learn to relax within 20 to 30 seconds in almost any situation—whether you're dealing with a difficult work situation, are caught in traffic, are starting to worry about your health, or are just unwinding in the middle of a hectic day. You'll also learn firsthand that the bodily sensations that you currently associate with disease are nothing but annoying by-products of the stress reaction and that *you* have the power to control them. Here we provide a description and detailed instructions for each of the three exercises. Practice each exercise for one week, in the order presented.

Week 1

The focus of the first week of practice is on what we call tense–release relaxation. You're going to need a quiet room, a comfortable chair, and 15 to 30 minutes of uninterrupted time during which you can do this once each day for the week. It's a good idea to try to set aside a regular time each day for practice, such as first thing in the morning, before supper, or at the end of the day. This helps make relaxation a part of your routine. It's also a good idea to reduce the chances of being interrupted. Turn off the ringer on the phone. Turn off your cell phone. Reduce background noise from other people by shutting the door and running a fan.

The purpose of tense–release relaxation is to train yourself to be more in tune with your body—to notice the difference between being tensed up and being relaxed. Muscle tension is a signal that your body is experiencing a stress reaction. The better you are at noticing tension, the better able you'll be to stop the stress reaction by using relaxation. You'll start by sitting in your chair and closing your eyes. Take off your shoes and loosen any tight clothing. Spend the first minute breathing deeply. Count to 6 while breathing in, and to 6 again while breathing out. Do this five or six times. While deep breathing, focus on your body and scan it for areas where you feel tension. Try to let the tension go. You'll notice that finding and letting go of muscle tension will get easier with practice. Now work through each of the muscle groups listed in Instruction Sheet 1. You need to tense the muscle for a count of 5, and then relax it for a count of 10. You'll do this two times for each muscle group. We don't want you to tense so hard that your muscles hurt or get cramped. If this happens, ease up a little. When relaxing the muscle, pay attention to the feelings in your body. It'll feel like the tension is draining off of your body. Once you've worked through all of the muscle groups, sit for another minute of deep breathing before you get up. Many people find it helpful to make themselves a tape recording of the instructions provided in Instruction Sheet 1 and to play it during practice. We recommend that you do this.

Week 2

After finishing week 1, you'll have become very good at noticing tension in your muscles. The next challenge is to learn how to relax without first having to tense your muscles. We call this release-only relaxation. You'll start this exercise just like week 1—sitting in a comfortable chair in a quiet room. Practice each

Instruction Sheet 1.
Tense–Release Relaxation Instructions

Today you're going to practice finding tension in your body. We'll start with some deep breathing, do some tensing and relaxing of muscle groups, and then finish with some more deep breathing. Please sit and adjust yourself so that you're comfortable. Now close your eyes. For the next minute or so you're going to do some deep breathing. When I say "inhale," breathe in for a count of 6. When I say "exhale,"breathe out for a count of 6. Breathe calm, regular breaths and feel how you relax more and more with each breath. While deep breathing, pay attention to your body and the way it feels. See if you can detect tension in any areas. Okay, ready?

Inhale, 2, 3, 4, 5, 6. Exhale, 2, 3, 4, 5, 6.
Inhale, 2, 3, 4, 5, 6. Exhale, 2, 3, 4, 5, 6.
Inhale, 2, 3, 4, 5, 6. Exhale, 2, 3, 4, 5, 6.
Inhale . . . . Exhale . . . .
Inhale . . . . Exhale . . . .
Inhale . . . . Exhale . . . .

Good. Now I'm going to have you practice tensing some groups of muscles for a count of 5, followed by relaxing the muscles for a count of 10. You'll do this two times for each muscle. I want you to breathe in when tensing your muscles and breathe out when relaxing. While relaxing your muscles also pay close attention to the feelings in your body. People describe the feelings differently and use different words. Most often, the feelings are described as a "draining off" or "emptying" of body tension. Let's begin.

Remember to breathe in while tensing. Breathe out while relaxing. Ready.

Clench your right hand into a fist. Hold it tight for a count of 5. Hold, 3, 4, 5. Now release and breathe out. Let your fingers relax. Can you feel tension draining off? Clench the same hand again. 1, 2, 3, 4, 5. Release. The tension should be flowing out of your hand.

Clench your left hand into a fist. Hold it tight for a count of 5. Hold, 3, 4, 5. Now release and breathe out. Let your fingers relax. Notice the tension draining off. Clench the same hand again. 1, 2, 3, 4, 5. Release. The tension should be flowing out of your hand.

Bend your right wrist in toward your forearm. Hold tight for a count of 5. Hold, 3, 4, 5. Now release and breathe out. Let your wrist relax. Feel the tension draining off. Now clench the same wrist again. 1, 2, 3, 4, 5. Release. The tension is now flowing off of your right wrist.

Bend your left wrist in toward your forearm. Hold tight for a count of 5. Hold, 3, 4, 5. Now release and breathe out. Let your wrist relax. Feel the tension draining off. Now clench the same wrist again. 1, 2, 3, 4, 5. Release. The tension is now flowing off of your left wrist.

(cont.)

Raise your right forearm and tense your bicep like a muscle man. Hold tight . . . and release . . . hold it tight again . . . and release. Feel the tension drain away.

Raise your left forearm and tense your bicep. Hold tight . . . and release . . . hold it tight again . . . and release. Feel the tension drain away.

Work through the following muscle groups in this same manner, holding tight while breathing in for a count of 5 and relaxing while exhaling slowly. If you're making a tape recording be sure to leave enough time for tensing and relaxing. It's not necessary at this point to put reminders on the tape to notice the tension draining but you can do so if you like. Remember to do the leg and toe exercises for both the right and left side of your body.

Shoulders	Raise shoulders toward ears.
Forehead	Raise eyebrows. Repeat this exercise while lowering eyebrows.
Eyes	Squint eyes (if you wear contact lenses, remove them before starting your practice session, or omit this muscle group).
Jaw	Push lower jaw outward.
Tongue	Push tongue against roof of mouth.
Throat	Yawn.
Neck	Gently rotate neck to the left. Repeat for right rotation, forward movement (chin to chest), and backward movement.
Chest	Take a deep breath and slowly exhale.
Upper back	Pull shoulders back and push chest outward.
Stomach	Push stomach outward. Repeat this exercise while pulling stomach all the way in.
Lower back	Arch lower back.
Legs I	Lock knee, point foot upward, and flex upper leg.
Legs II	Lock knee, point foot outward, and flex upper leg.
Toes I	Curl toes down.
Toes II	Curl toes upward.

Excellent! Now take a minute to enjoy your relaxed state.

Inhale, 2, 3, 4, 5, 6. Exhale, 2, 3, 4, 5, 6.
Inhale . . . . . .Exhale . . . .
Inhale . . . . . .Exhale . . . .
Inhale . . . . . .Exhale . . . .
Inhale . . . . . .Exhale . . . .

You're done for today.

day of the week, two times per day, for about 10 minutes. Close your eyes and breathe deeply for a minute or so at the start. This week we want you to say "relax" under your breath each time you breathe out. Continue breathing deeply for another five minutes while scanning your body for muscle tension. Go over each muscle group, starting with your face and moving down through your neck, chest, upper back, arms, hands, stomach, lower back, and legs and ending at your feet and toes. When you find areas of tension, try to let the tension go. Release it! If need be, you can tense the muscle briefly before releasing. Remember to repeat the word "relax" quietly to yourself each time you breathe out. This trains you to link the word "relax" with relaxation of each muscle group. Do this for about 5 minutes. You can use the instructions in Instruction Sheet 2 to make a tape recording to play during practice. If you do use a tape recording, we want you to fade it out and do the release-only relaxation exercise without it by the end of day 4.

Week 3

The tense–release and release-only relaxation exercises teach you how to find tension in your body and put a stop to it. The week 3 exercises—what we call *rapid relaxation*—will make your newfound relaxation skills fast acting and portable. The goal is to relax within 20 to 30 seconds, anytime, anywhere; not just when sitting in a comfortable chair in a quiet room. There are three steps to rapid relaxation:

1. Take three deep breaths, inhaling and exhaling slowly.
2. Repeat the word "relax" to yourself while exhaling.
3. Scan your entire body quickly for tension and release it as much as possible while exhaling.

You can start practicing rapid relaxation while in your quiet room, seated in your comfortable chair. A tape recording isn't necessary or recommended at this stage. Work through the three steps. This should take about 30 seconds. Repeat the three steps about 20 times in a row for each of days 1 and 2. Once you feel you've got it down, move outside of your quiet room and practice while seated in other rooms of your home. On days 3 and 4 you can begin practicing while standing or walking, releasing tension in all the muscles that aren't involved in these activities. For example, your legs and lower back will have some natural tension to maintain your posture when you're standing, but you should be able to relax your face, neck, shoulders, arms, hands, and so forth. Run through the three steps until you feel relaxed.

You need to do the rapid relaxation about 20 times per day for days 3 through 7. Use days 5 through 7 to practice in more challenging situations. These might include while sitting in traffic, standing in a line, taking a stressful

Instruction Sheet 2.
Release-Only Relaxation Instructions

Today you're going to relax without tensing your muscles first. Start with some deep breathing, scan your body from head to toe for tension, and relax while deep breathing. When you breathe out say the word "relax" quietly under your breath. Do this each time you breathe out. Are you sitting comfortably? Then we'll begin.

Breathe with calm, regular breaths and feel how you relax more and more with each breath. Let go and relax. Inhale, 2, 3, 4, 5, 6. Exhale. Remember to say the word "relax" quietly under your breath as you breathe out. Inhale, 2, 3, 4, 5, 6. Exhale, 2, 3, 4, 5, 6. Inhale . . . . . Exhale . . . . . Inhale . . . . . Exhale . . . . . Inhale . . . . . Exhale. Continue saying the word "relax" each time you breathe out. Now relax your forehead . . . Eyelids . . . Jaw . . . Tongue . . . Throat . . . Your entire face. Repeat the word "relax" each time you breathe out. Relax your neck . . . Shoulders . . . Arms . . . Chest . . . Upper back. Continue saying the word "relax" each time you breathe out. Breathe with calm, regular breaths. Let the relaxation spread down to your stomach . . . Lower back . . . Thighs . . . Calves . . . Out the tips of your toes. Say the word "relax" each time you breathe out. Inhale . . . Exhale . . . Feel your relaxation deepen with every breath you take. Take a deep breath and hold it for a couple of seconds . . . Let the air out slowly. Notice how you relax more and more. Take another deep breath and hold it . . . . Exhale. Now open your eyes.

Are you feeling relaxed?

phone call, or getting supper ready. At the completion of week 3 you'll be able to relax quickly and in almost any situation. You'll have trained yourself to relax whenever you slowly exhale and say "relax." (Some people find it helpful to leave themselves reminders to practice rapid relaxation. You might try putting a note on your computer monitor or a colored sticky dot on your watch, cell phone, or rearview mirror.)

Things to Remember

These exercises will teach you that the stress reaction is something you can control. By taking a minute to relax when things start getting hectic, you'll stop your sympathetic nervous system from preparing for "fight or flight." If you practice consistently over the next three weeks, we guarantee you'll feel a difference. If you want to "see" the difference, do the following. Using Worksheet 3, rate the stress-related bodily sensations you've experienced and how bothersome they've been over the week just before starting the relaxation exercises. Repeat these ratings at the end of weeks 1, 2, and 3. At the end of week 3 you can review your ratings, looking at the number of bodily sensations you experienced over each week, as well as how bothersome they were. An example is shown in Figure 3. Notice that although neither of Garth's bodily sensations went away completely, the amount of discomfort they caused him decreased quite a bit.

These exercises will also teach you that many of the bodily sensations you experience are annoying by-products of being stressed out. Like a light controlled

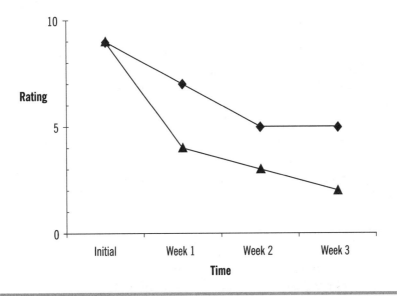

FIGURE 3. **Garth's ratings of distress from stomach cramps (diamonds) and aches and pains (triangles) before and during applied relaxation training.**

by a switch, you can turn them off at will. They're *not* signs or symptoms of disease. These are important lessons that may dramatically affect you by reducing your health anxiety. The message we want you to get out of these exercises is

> "The sensations I once feared as being part of some disease process are, in fact, nothing but harmless by-products of the stress reaction that are under my control,"

not

> "I'm afraid these sensations are telling me something's wrong with my body. They're not harmless. But I can avoid experiencing them if I use relaxation."

It's okay if, at the end of week 3, you find that your feelings are more in line with this second message. This isn't uncommon. The exercises in Chapter 6 are designed to move you toward feeling in line with the first message.

Retraining Your Breathing Patterns: Weeks 4 and 5

Some people, particularly those with anxiety disorders and health anxiety, breathe too much. Without knowing it, they're almost always hyperventilating. That is, they breathe by taking short, shallow breaths, usually with their chests. This happens naturally when faced with stressors and, as you might have guessed, is part of the sympathetic nervous system preparations for "fight or flight." It becomes a problem when you breathe like this all the time. Why? Although harmless, this type of breathing keeps us on edge and isn't conducive to relaxation. That's why we started our relaxation exercises with deep breathing. This type of breathing also reduces the amount of oxygen circulating in the bloodstream, causing dizziness and light-headedness, and strains the chest muscles, causing chest pain. These may be some of the sensations that cause you concern. By retraining yourself to breathe more deeply and with your diaphragm (the muscle that lies between your stomach and base of your lungs), you can achieve a more relaxed state and gain control over those annoying, harmless bodily sensations.

How are you breathing right now? Are your breaths rapid and shallow? Do they seem to be centered in your chest? Is your chest moving more than your stomach area? Do you often feel short of breath? Do you yawn or sigh a lot? If you answered *yes* to several of these questions, you'll likely benefit from our breathing retraining exercise. With consistent practice, you'll eventually breathe more deeply and with your diaphragm without even thinking about it. Breathing retraining takes about two weeks and should be done during the fourth and fifth week of your practice.

Week 4

Breathing retraining is rather simple. First, you need to see the difference between chest breathing and diaphragm breathing. To do so, place one hand on your chest and the other on your stomach. Now take a breath in through your nose, moving the air to the top of your lungs. Keep your stomach still. You'll feel your ribcage move upward and outward. You'll also feel tension in your upper chest. Breathe out through your mouth, letting your rib-cage move inward and downward. Do this a few times. This is what chest breathing feels like. Now breathe through your nose, moving the air to the bottom of your lungs. Keep your chest still. Your stomach will move outward. Breathe out slowly through your mouth. You'll notice the feeling of a slight downward movement in your stomach area while exhaling. Do this a few times. This is diaphragm breathing.

Practice alternating between chest breathing and diaphragm breathing until you can tell the difference. Next you'll practice the diaphragm breathing for about 10 minutes. Make yourself comfortable, either lying or sitting in a quiet space. Breathe in slowly through your nose for a count of 2, pause for a count of 1 or 2, and let the air flow out slowly as you exhale for a count of 2. Be certain to feel your stomach rising and falling with each breath. Don't move your chest. Your breathing should be intentional and comfortable. Using these instructions, you'll be breathing at a rate of 10 to 12 breaths per minute. You can slow things down by adding an extra second to the inhalations and exhalations. We want you to practice this twice a day for a week. You can make a tape recording to help pace your breathing during practice, saying "in" for two seconds, pausing for one or two seconds, and saying "out" for two seconds. If you make a tape recording, use it for the first five minutes of practice and complete the final five minutes without it.

Week 5

With consistent practice during week 4, you'll quickly become proficient at diaphragm breathing. During week 5 we want you to practice diaphragm breathing in everyday situations. You can practice while reading (in fact, do it while reading the next few chapters), watching TV, waiting in line, sitting in traffic, and so on. You can gradually start practicing in more hectic situations, much like with the relaxation exercises.

Things to Remember

Retraining yourself to breathe with your diaphragm will have several positive effects. It'll activate the parasympathetic nervous system and thereby put your body in a relaxed "business-as-usual" state. You'll feel less keyed up. When you notice your breathing becoming shallower and focused in your chest, signaling the onset of a stress reaction, you'll be able to gain control by practicing diaphragm breathing. Combining diaphragm breathing with rapid relaxation will give you considerable control over the way you (and your body) respond to stressors.

Problem-Solving Skills: Week 6

Every day we're faced with problems that require solutions: deciding how to finish a work or school assignment on time; fixing a problem with the computer; finding a partner; whether to go away for the weekend with the family or stay home and get caught up on work; finding money to pay this month's bills; settling a disagreement with a family member. The list goes on and on.

Solving life's problems can be challenging and, yes, stressful. Our relaxation and breathing retraining exercises teach you to control the stress reaction. But you can also learn skills that will improve your success in solving problems. We recommend a 12-step program for problem solving. The main objectives of the program are to:

- Pick specific problems to focus on,
- Identify and set your goals,
- Tackle the steps needed to attain the set goals, and
- Review your progress.

The 12 steps are outlined on Worksheet 4. You can work through these steps for any problem you face, whether it's simple or very complicated. As with the relaxation and breathing retraining exercises, regular daily practice makes perfect! We recommend that you identify a simple problem and spend week 6 practicing ways of solving it. For example, you might try to solve the problem of which of two TV programs that are on at the same time to watch. Work toward more complicated or urgent problems, such as resolving conflicts with loved ones or finding a dating partner. Devote week 6 to problem-solving practice. Use the skills you learn to deal with and overcome the day-to-day problems you encounter.

If you're finding it hard to find time to spend on working through the exercises in this book, you might try working through the steps to overcome the things that are getting in your way. Maureen was finding it hard to practice because she had to work all day, rush home to get supper ready for everybody, run the kids to their activities, and then get them ready for bed. She worked through the steps with her husband and came up with a "divide and conquer" solution— they would alternate nights cooking and chauffeuring the kids around in order to free up a few of Maureen's evenings. Paul was able to gain an hour every evening by cutting back the time he spent surfing the Internet. He spent half of this time practicing and the other half playing with his six-year-old daughter. Reward

Worksheet 4. A 12-Step Approach to Problem Solving

There are solutions to most of life's problems. The chances of effectively solving your problems depend on the approach you take. The following steps increase the chances of solving important problems in your life.

1. **Pick a problem** that you would like to work on. It could be a big, urgent problem that may take some effort to solve, or it might be a little one. Successfully tackling small problems can increase your confidence of solving bigger problems. List your problem as specifically as possible:

   _____

2. **State your goal.** Please be as specific as possible. What is the outcome that you are hoping to attain? For example, if you are an unemployed accountant, your goal might be to find a full-time accounting position.

   _____

   _____

   _____

3. **Is your goal realistic?** If not, list another, more attainable goal.

   _____

4. **What are your resources for attaining your goal?** This would include material resources (for example, money, transportation) and social resources (for example, people who could help you or offer support).

   _____

   _____

   _____

5. **Brainstorm!** List all the possible ways of attaining your goal that you can think of. List these possibilities regardless of whether they're plausible or not. Use an extra sheet if necessary.

   _____

   _____

   _____

6. **Refine your solutions.** Look through your list of solutions and see if you can think of ways of improving your solutions. If you think of extra solutions while doing this, then write them down as well.

   _____

   _____

   _____

(cont.)

7. **Evaluate.** List the pros and cons of each solution. Which one looks the best?

_____

_____

_____

_____

8. **Baby steps.** Can you break your goal up into subgoals? For example, if your goal was to find a dating partner, your subgoals might be the following: (a) Put yourself in situations in which you will meet people whom you might like to date (for example, join a sporting club or enroll in a course at a community center). (b) Get to know people. Make friends. Even if you don't find a dating partner, at least you'll have friends. (c) If you find someone attractive, arrange to have coffee with him or her . . . and so on.

_____

_____

_____

_____

9. **Identify obstacles.** What are the things that might get in the way of solving your problems? These might be behavioral obstacles (for example, lack of job skills) or thinking obstacles (for example, negative thoughts such as "Nobody would ever hire me."). List your obstacles here.

_____

_____

_____

_____

10. **Overcome your roadblocks.** List ways of overcoming the obstacles. This might involve improving your skills or challenging your negative thoughts.

_____

_____

_____

_____

11. **Make a commitment** to solving your problems. Plan to do something each day.

12. **Track your progress** toward achieving your goals. Are you making steady progress? If so, good. If not, then identify the roadblocks and try to come up with solutions. Sometimes it helps to reward yourself for your efforts in overcoming problems, especially big problems. Treat yourself to something nice.

Source: Adapted from S. Taylor and G. J. G. Asmundson (2004). *Treating health anxiety: A cognitive-behavioral approach.* New York: Guilford Press. Adapted by permission.

yourself for consistent efforts at working through the 12 steps of successful problem solving. It takes work, but it feels great to overcome life's obstacles.

Time Management: Week 7

We're firm believers in leading a balanced life. This means finding time for work, family, leisure, and yourself. It also means keeping that sympathetic nervous system in check and allowing the business-as-usual functions of the parasympathetic nervous system to operate. A tall order in today's hectic world! Make it a priority in your life to find balance.

A helpful strategy to finding balance that builds on relaxation, breathing, and problem solving is time management. Poor time management usually leads a person to feel overwhelmed and stressed out. Ask yourself the following questions:

- Am I often rushing from one activity to another?
- Am I frequently running late?
- Is my productivity low?
- Do I have trouble finishing important tasks?

If you answered *yes* to one or more of these questions, then you likely have poor time-management skills. There are many excellent resources that can assist you in becoming proficient with organizing and getting the most from the hours in your day. We've listed several resources in the Resources section at the back of this book. Working through the steps of successful problem solving can also help with managing your time. A simplified approach to time management involves the following steps and can be practiced during week 7.

- *Create a weekly "to-do" list.* Decide what you want to accomplish for the week and write it down. Look forward. Make a long-range list that covers the next month.
- *Set priorities.* Rate the priority of the things on your "to do" list. Which are high priority and need to be done now? Which are medium priority? Which can wait or be given up? In today's world it's almost impossible to get everything done. It's okay to give some things up.
- *Estimate time requirements and set a regular schedule.* Be frank in determining how long it will take to complete tasks. Use a day planner to set aside regular "appointments" to work on a specific task and work on that task during the appointment. Also, if possible, don't allow your appointment to be interrupted. Turn off your e-mail, don't answer the phone, and put a "do not disturb" sign on your door before closing it. When possible, try to finish one task rather than jumping back and forth between several tasks. These strategies will increase the likelihood that you'll get done.

• *Match the task to your energy level.* If you're a morning person, schedule your appointments for working on tasks in the morning when your energy is highest. Do likewise if you're an afternoon or evening person. Don't schedule appointments for times when you know you're usually tired.

• *Be honest about what you can handle.* Most people have more tasks at work and at home than they can handle. If you're overcommitted, don't be afraid to say *no* to a request (sometimes this isn't possible, but in many cases it is). Are there things you can get someone else to do? For example, your spouse or a friend could take your daughter to swimming lessons, and your office mate might take on part of an assignment. Are there ways of doing things more efficiently? Things rarely need to be perfect.

• *Are you a procrastinator?* Procrastinators realize that things need to be done, but they keep putting them off. People often put off doing things because they overestimate the difficulty of a task and underestimate their ability to suc-cessfully complete the task. If you're doing this, try using your day planner to set an appointment, and work on the task whether you feel like it or not. Chances are that once you get started, you'll want to continue. Motivate yourself by treat-ing yourself to something you like once a task is completed.

Good time-management skills are particularly important for people with health anxiety. First, these skills build on those of relaxation, diaphragm breath-ing, and successful problem solving by promoting a generally less stressful life. Second, they help prioritize important work, family, and personal leisure activi-ties—things that when given proper attention make us feel good about our-selves—and downgrade the importance of spending a lot of time checking vari-ous information sources about bodily sensations or seeking reassurance from others. Checking and reassurance seeking have low priority relative to your fam-ily, work, and personal leisure and, in fact, are counterproductive to breaking the anxiety cycle.

Practice Is Important

Acknowledging the possibility that the things you currently view as signs and symptom of disease are harmless by-products of your body's stress reaction is the starting point to conquering your health anxiety. Setting aside scheduled appointments with yourself to work on our strategies will allow you ample opportunity to take back your life and live it. Practicing relaxation, retraining your breathing, improving your problem-solving skills, and becoming a good manager of your time will have a generally positive effect on your life. Over the next seven weeks it will become much less hectic. You'll feel more in control. These skills may also have a significant impact on your health anxiety. By work-ing hard at controlling the stress reaction, you'll learn for yourself that many of the bodily sensations that you once associated with disease are, in fact, under *your* control.

Where to Now?

We've mentioned several times already that our strategies can help you overcome your health anxiety and get back to living life to its fullest. How motivated and interested were you in trying out our strategies at the beginning of the chapter? How about now that you've tried our approach to stress management? Were we successful in showing you that you can control the stress responses of your body and, in doing so, provide some relief from the unwanted and anxiety-provoking bodily sensations that you experience? Are you willing to give our strategies a chance to make a *significant* change in your life? If your answer is *yes* to these questions, you're ready to move on to some strategies that specifically target some of the thoughts and behaviors that feed your health anxiety.

Gunnar was very skeptical when first introduced to our program. In fact, his initial thought was that it was a bunch of rubbish: "Pain is my problem, not anxiety!" His son encouraged him to read through the material and give it a shot, reminding him that nothing else seemed to be working. Gunnar noticed how much less severe his pain was when he used relaxation and time-management strategies. Within a few weeks he'd developed a new perspective about his pain:

> "I learned a whole new approach for dealing with a seven-year, twenty-four-hour-a-day curse that hadn't occurred to me before. Suddenly my universe shifted."

He was able to take back some of the control over his life that he'd lost to pain.

Six

Thoughts That Influence Your Anxiety and How to Change Them

The way you think about noise in your body plays a big role in the way you view your health and the way you feel. That's the reason we're going to spend some time on your thoughts. Just as you've learned to identify tension in your body and take control of it through relaxation, you'll learn to make changes to your anxiety-inducing thinking patterns, which will help break the health anxiety cycle. In fact, the relaxation practice you've been doing may have already affected the way you think about some bodily sensations you experience. Did the stress management exercises you've been practicing help you see firsthand that some of your bodily sensations are related to the stress reaction? Are you now better able to control them? Do you feel less anxious about them? If you answered *yes* to these questions, you're making excellent progress. If you answered *no*, don't despair! All the people we see in therapy progress at different rates. Self-help strategies are no different. While reading through this chapter, keep practicing the stress management exercises outlined in Chapter 5. Further exploration of how you think about your health may be what's needed to break your health anxiety cycle.

We're *not* suggesting that what you're experiencing is "all in your head." Your bodily sensations and your concerns about them are real. However, the way you think about them—your cognitions—can make them seem more harmful to your physical well-being than they really are. The word *cognition* refers to many of the concepts we introduced in Chapter 2—beliefs, assumptions, perception, attention, and interpretation (or misinterpretation)—as well as other mental processes related to thinking. Cognitive-behavioral therapists are interested in helping people reduce their anxiety by changing their anxiety-provoking thoughts. The goal for people with too much health anxiety is to change beliefs, assumptions, and interpretations (or what we'll call *specific thoughts* for short) that keep alive the idea that bodily sensations can be explained only by disease. In the case of people with disease phobia, the goal is to challenge the notion that they're destined to catch some horrific disease. In this chapter we'll help you work toward breaking your anxiety cycle by teaching you:

- To be more aware of any specific thoughts about bodily sensations and vulnerability to disease that cause you to worry too much about your health, and
- How to replace these with alternative (and possibly more accurate) ways of thinking about your concerns that aren't so anxiety provoking.

We'll do this by helping you figure out *how you think* about your health and *what you think* about your health (week 8). Then we'll teach you a number of strategies for changing the specific thoughts that make you anxious about your health (weeks 9 and 10).

How You Think about Your Health: Week 8

We've given you several examples of the kinds of specific thoughts that people with health anxiety have. Jonathan (see Chapter 1) was pretty sure that recent sluggishness and pain in his legs was the result of undiagnosed multiple sclerosis or a brain tumor. Sarah (see Chapter 1) concluded that her breast lumps must be cancerous because the Mayo Clinic doctors found cancer in an acquaintance of hers who'd been told by other doctors that nothing was wrong. Bob (see Chapter 1) believed that wearing latex gloves would protect him from the germs lurking on door handles and in public washrooms. All of these people have in common the fact that they think about the changes and sensations they experience in their bodies in unhelpful ways. One of the unhelpful beliefs you might have held before working through Chapter 5 is that noise in your body is almost always a sign or symptom of disease. You've already learned that some bodily sensations are part of the stress reaction, and as a result your ways of thinking about your health may have already changed a bit. But it's likely that you have some more specific ways of thinking about your health that you might not even be aware of that feed your health anxiety.

People don't usually give much thought to how they think about things. We often have to learn how to think this way. You'll need to learn to spot the ways of thinking that make your health anxiety worse. Believing that a single occurrence of a symptom is proof of having a disease (called *overgeneralized thinking*) and thinking that something is physically wrong because you feel "down in the dumps" (called *emotional reasoning*) are very common. Most people over-generalize and use emotional reasoning when thinking about changes and sensations in their bodies that they believe to be symptoms of disease. These ways of thinking are often (but not always) easy to identify and are usually easier to overcome than some of the other ways of thinking that we describe here. This makes them an excellent starting point for teaching you to understand how the way you think about your health can make your health anxiety worse.

Here are some examples of the overgeneralizations that people make. Some are fairly general, not being related to any particular disease, and others are very specific. The last few are more characteristic of people with disease phobia.

- "It hurts so bad, there must be something seriously wrong with me."
- "I've been so tired lately, I must be really sick."
- "I can't stop peeing. I must have diabetes."
- "What's this pain in my head? I must have a brain tumor."
- "My groin won't stop hurting. I bet I have an ectopic pregnancy."
- "I've been so sluggish this week. It must be multiple sclerosis."
- "I've never felt light-headed like this before. I bet a blood vessel in my brain is just waiting to explode."
- "This stiffness in my knuckles must be a sign of arthritis."
- "My bowels are going nuts. I've got diarrhea. Sometimes there's blood when I wipe and my butt's leaking into my shorts. It must be colitis or maybe even rectal cancer."
- "These night sweats are weird. I've read that people with Hodgkin's disease have night sweats. I must have Hodgkin's."
- "The skin on my foot is itchy and doesn't look right. I think it's flesh-eating disease."
- "I can't go near sick people. I'll catch what they've got and then I'll die."
- "Doors and doorknobs are covered in germs. If I touch them I'll catch something."

Can you relate to any of these examples or something like them? Be honest with yourself, keeping in mind that everyone makes overgeneralizations. You might feel embarrassed or uncomfortable viewing yourself in this way. But being honest with yourself is a necessary part of changing your ways of thinking about your health. Take a few minutes to write down any thoughts you've had in the recent past that fit this pattern in the *overgeneralization* column of Worksheet 5. We've noticed that this exercise is easier to complete if you start by listing symptoms (for example, racing heart or headache) or situations (for example, using a public washroom or being around sick people) and then deciding if you've made overgeneralizations about each one.

Worksheet 5.
Identifying Overgeneralizations and Emotional Reasoning

Symptom/situation	Overgeneralization
Headache	This headache means I must have a brain tumor.
Touching doorknobs	If I touch doorknobs, I'll catch some nasty infectious disease.

Your feelings	Emotional reasoning
Anxious and on edge	I must be sick, otherwise I wouldn't feel so anxious.

We also want you to think about times when you've assumed you're sick because you're feeling down in the dumps or anxious. Some examples are such thoughts as "There must be something wrong with me; otherwise I wouldn't be so on edge"; "I'm feeling so sad. I must be ill"; and "I wouldn't be feeling so emotional if I wasn't sick." Have you had thoughts like these? Write down an example of having taken your feelings as evidence of being sick in the *emotional reasoning* column of Worksheet 5. As with the overgeneralizations, this exercise is easier if you start with a negative emotion you've had and think about whether you've linked it to your health in some way.

Try to write down at least one example each of overgeneralization and emotional reasoning. If you have difficulty, don't despair. We all have these kinds of thoughts, but sometimes people can become less aware of thoughts they have on a regular basis. You might need to monitor your past and present thoughts about your health in order to recognize generalizations and emotional reasoning. To do this you can simply watch for bodily sensations or strong emotions you feel over the next few days and jot down the first few thoughts that come to mind upon noticing the sensations or emotions. The purpose of this exercise is to help you start becoming more aware of the thoughts you have about your health.

Being able to identify generalizations and emotional reasoning is an important step in learning how you think about your health. It will help you identify more specific ways of thinking that may be helping to keep your health anxiety alive. These include *all-or-none thinking, negatively biased thinking, jumping to catastrophic conclusions, selective attention,* and *superstitious thinking*. The next step is to figure out which of these ways of thinking apply to you. By giving honest answers to the following items, you'll be able understand your ways of thinking. If you're having difficulty responding to any of the items—perhaps avoiding a *yes* response while not being entirely certain that the answer is no—try listing the types of thoughts you have whenever faced with the symptoms and situations you fear. This will help you come up with answers.

All-or-None Thinking

- I'm either healthy or seriously ill. There's no in-between.

  Yes   No

- Medical tests are worthless if they're not 100 percent accurate.

  Yes   No

- I need to be completely certain that I'm healthy.

  Yes   No

If you answered *yes* to any of these questions, you have what is called *all-or-none thinking*. This is a type of thinking by which you see things as either black or white. You don't leave any room for the many shades of gray that can fall between the two extremes. People who have an all-or-none way of thinking are also usually unwilling to accept any uncertainty; things either are or they aren't.

Negatively Biased Thinking

- I focus on negative information about my health and tend to overlook or ignore the positive things. (Example: "I usually don't remember much of what I hear or read about hopeful medical advances, but I always remember the negative information.")

  Yes   No

- I'm usually unwilling to believe positive information about my health. (Example: "I usually feel uneasy when I leave my doctor's office having gotten nothing but good news. I feel I haven't gotten the whole story or that my doc has missed something.")

  Yes   No

If you answered *yes* to either of these questions, you have what we call *negatively biased thinking*. People with negatively biased thinking tend to pick out a single negative point and ignore all the positives about their health. They also don't want to accept positive information about their health at face value. Jonathan's family doctor told him that because the specialist had ruled out neurological conditions and cancer he probably had nothing to worry about. Rather than viewing this as a good thing, Jonathan focused on the word *probably*. He interpreted this as meaning there was still uncertainty about his health and spent a lot of time thinking about other deadly causes for his symptoms. In a similar manner, Joan insisted that test findings indicating she didn't have cancer "don't count" because they might be wrong.

Jumping to Catastrophic Conclusions

- I worry that any "noise" in my body means that something's seriously wrong with my health.

  Yes   No

- I always expect the worst when waiting for the results of a medical exam or test that I've had.

  Yes   No

- I often think that I'll never recover if I get a serious disease

  Yes   No

Answering *yes* to any of these questions indicates that you have a tendency to *jump to catastrophic conclusions* when thinking about your health. We all go through a process of self-diagnosis when we notice bodily sensations that are thought to be signs or symptoms of disease. We ask ourselves, "What's going on in my body?" and "Could I be sick?" People with health anxiety tend to quickly conclude that they're sick without taking enough time to consider other possible explanations for the bodily sensations or to weigh the evidence for and against the conclusion that they're sick. Many of our patients jump to the worst possible or most catastrophic conclusions, such as that a headache must be a symptom of an undiagnosed brain tumor, a breast lump must be a sign of cancer, chest pain must indicate a serious heart problem, upset stomach must be an ulcer or even something worse, and so on.

Selective Attention

- I'm more sensitive to bodily sensations and changes in my body than most people.

Yes   No

- I experience more pain and other unpleasant bodily sensations than most people.

Yes   No

- It's hard for me to focus on anything but my health and whether I'm sick.

Yes   No

If you answered *yes* to any of these questions, you have what we described in Chapter 2 as *selective attention*. This is a style of thinking by which attention is focused inward on sensations and changes in your body that you believe are related to disease. It increases your chances of false alarms and often increases negatively biased thinking and jumping to catastrophic conclusions. For example, John was so worried that he'd have a heart attack that he watched for any signs that this might happen. He didn't notice any big fluctuations in his heart rate, but when he awoke with sore ribs he immediately concluded that he was having a heart attack and rushed to the emergency room. Despite the doctors telling him he had the heart of a race horse and that nothing seemed to be wrong, he was unwilling to accept this and was convinced the doctor was wrong. He went home and continued to watch for signs of an oncoming heart attack.

Superstitious Thinking

Some of our patients have told us things such as

"I've been taking garlic pills every day for years and haven't had any heart problems. The garlic pills protect me from getting heart disease and having a heart attack"

and

"I stay away from hospitals. I've done this for years and haven't caught any nasty diseases. It's because I stay away from hospitals."

Does this sound at all like you? Do you assume that something you do prevents bad things from happening because the bad event hasn't happened so far? This is called *superstitious thinking*. It's akin to believing that garlic cloves ward off vampires ("I carry garlic cloves with me and I've never seen a vampire. Therefore the cloves must be working"). Many people with health anxiety have superstitious thoughts that contribute to their health anxiety.

Helpful Hint

You need to know how you think about your health in order to change the way you think about it. Giving frank answers to the preceding items will help you discover how you think about your health. Put a check mark in the blank beside each of the ways of thinking that apply to you.

_____ All-or-none thinking
_____ Negatively biased thinking
___✓___ Jumping to catastrophic conclusions
_____ Selective attention
_____ Superstitious thinking

The way you think is closely related to what you think. You'll be well prepared for the next section if you've completed the week 8 exercises and questions before moving on.

What You Think about Your Health

You can't change ways of thinking that increase health anxiety without being crystal clear about your thoughts about health and disease. You need to put your finger on exactly what your specific thoughts are. You've already started this process by writing down examples of your overgeneralizations and emotional reasoning about health on Worksheet 5 and by figuring out your ways of thinking about health. Working through the following exercise will help you do this in more depth.

Take a few minutes now to think about a recent episode of health anxiety that you've had. For example, how the piercing head pain you've been experiencing over the past few days has caused you to worry that you have a brain tumor, or how you've been prodding and probing a lump under your skin that you fear is cancerous. Describe the details of the episode on Worksheet 6. Write down the sequence of events that occurred during the episode—the sensations or changes in your body, your thoughts, your feelings, and what you did to make

Worksheet 6.
Details of a Recent Health Anxiety Episode

One of My Recent Episodes of Health Anxiety

it through the episode. Put in as much detail as you can. Don't evaluate whether some part of what happened was good or bad, just describe it. If you've had episodes that are related to different worries—for example, times that you worry you've got cancer and other times when you worry you've got multiple sclerosis—you might want to write down the details for each. It should take you about 10 minutes to work through this exercise.

Now answer the following questions about the example or examples you provided.

- What was the most upsetting thing about this? What were you most worried about?
- How would you react if your main worry came true? How would you feel? What would you do?
- What's the worst that could happen if your worry came true? How would this affect your life?
- What would a person who knew little about you think about this?

Your answers to these questions will give you an idea of your specific thoughts—your beliefs, assumptions, perceptions, and interpretations—that help maintain your health anxiety. Do any of your thoughts fit into any of the ways of thinking we described earlier? These specific thoughts will become targets for change.

Before moving on to strategies for changing your specific thoughts, we're going to have you track details of any episodes of health anxiety that you have over the next few weeks. We call this *prospective monitoring*. The benefit of prospective monitoring is that it lets you collect very specific information about your thoughts and feelings during bouts of health anxiety that you haven't yet experienced. You can use Worksheet 7 to write down important details of the episodes you have. Make copies so you have enough space for keeping track of all episodes that happen over the next 14 days. (Use a longer time frame if you're not overly anxious during this time.) In particular, we want you to note when the episode occurred, what triggered it, the specific thought you had at the time, how convincing your thought was, and how much anxiety you were feeling. Also, in preparation for some of the strategies we'll present to you in Chapter 7, we want you to make note of what you did to deal with your worry and anxiety (without evaluating whether or not this was a good or bad thing to do). An example of how much information to write down is provided on the worksheet and should help you get started.

Helpful Hint

If you find you're having difficulty filling out Worksheets 6 and 7, you can re-review the material presented in Chapter 2 and the "How You Think about Your Health" section in this chapter. Ask yourself, "Do any of the examples sound

Worksheet 7. Health Anxiety Thoughts and Behaviors Monitoring Form

Day and date	Health anxiety trigger (for example, an event or bodily sensation)	Specific thoughts (and strength of belief from 0 to 100 percent)	Intensity of anxiety (0–100)	What you did to deal with your anxiety.
Tuesday at 6:35 p.m.	Saw a TV program on breast cancer.	Worried that small lumps in my breasts were cancerous. (Believed it 100 percent.)	95	Checked my body for more lumps. Checked so much that my breasts were tender and sore.

Source. Adapted from S. Taylor and G. J. G. Asmundson (2004). *Treating health anxiety: A cognitive-behavioral approach.* New York: Guilford Press. Adapted by permission.

like me?" and "Am I doing things similar to the people in the examples?" Reflecting on your own thoughts and behaviors, especially when they've become a core feature of who "you" are, is a challenging task. You can also look back over Worksheet 1 in Chapter 2, where you made notes on some of your symptoms and initial thoughts about them. Another helpful strategy is to try taking another person's perspective. That is, try to imagine what an outside viewer of you, your thoughts, and your behaviors would "see." Or you might try thinking about how you'd respond to a friend in a similar situation. This strategy works because it's easier to make objective evaluations when you get away from the emotions involved with the situation. If you take a step-by-step approach, completing the worksheets in order, we're confident in your ability to successfully identify specific thoughts you have about your health.

Ridding Yourself of Anxiety-Inducing Thoughts: Weeks 9 and 10

At this point you should be armed with a good understanding of (1) the ways of thinking that characterize you when thinking about your health, (2) the specific thoughts you have about your health, (3) how strongly you believe in these thoughts, and (4) how much anxiety they cause. This is a very important step in taking back control of your life. Well done! You're now ready to begin work on replacing your anxiety-provoking thoughts with thoughts that are less anxiety provoking and that more accurately reflect what is known about the diseases you fear having. Strategies for doing this include examining the evidence for and against your disease-related thoughts, challenging the need for certainty, taking another person's perspective, evaluating the "cost" of your beliefs, and attention focusing.

Here we describe each of these strategies and provide some exercises that will allow you to try them out. We recommend that you read through all of the strategies and follow our suggestions as you go along. However, don't spend too much time practicing any one strategy until you've finished reading about each of them. Some of the strategies may be better suited to you than others. This will depend, to some extent, on your patterns of thinking. It will also depend on which strategy or strategies you like using the best. If one seems to be working better than the others, stick with it.

Playing Medical Detective: Examining the Evidence

Throughout this chapter we've been suggesting that there are ways of thinking about your signs and symptoms that are more anxiety provoking than others. You can take our word for it if you like, or you can gather your own evidence and test our suggestions for yourself. This can be a very effective strategy for changing ways of thinking that increase health anxiety. Our patients learn how to do this by using Worksheet 8. The strategy involves a few basic steps:

- Collect evidence *for* the accuracy of a specific thought,
- Collect evidence *against* the accuracy of a specific thought, and
- Consider whether there are other ways of looking at the situation.

You might find this difficult at first because up until now you've probably been considering only evidence that supports the idea that you're sick. Let's look at an example and break it down so that you can try for yourself.

At the beginning of Chapter 1 we introduced you to Joan, a 44-year-old director of finance in a growing company and single mother of a young son. She had been experiencing stomach upset, nausea, bloating, and pain for about a month. Several doctors told her that nothing was wrong physically and that the cause was likely diet or stress. Not buying this explanation, Joan became extremely worried that she had terminal stomach cancer. She completed all of the exercises described here and, using Worksheet 7, noted the specific thought that her stomach upset and related symptoms were the result of stomach cancer. She believed this with 97 percent certainty, and she rated her anxiety intensity at 90 percent. We asked Joan to take on the role of medical detective to (1) find evidence for this specific thought, (2) find evidence against it, and (3) come up with one or more alternate, noncatastrophic explanations that could also be evaluated. Her completed Worksheet 8 is shown in Figure 4.

Joan learned several important things in working through this exercise. First, she recognized that there was evidence *against* her belief that she had stomach cancer. Second, she realized that she'd been so wrapped up in thinking she had cancer that she'd never even stopped to think about other noncatastrophic and non-disease-based explanations for her stomach discomfort. In the end she was able to come up with an alternate explanation that she could accept—that her stomach upset was from pushing too hard at work and being emotionally exhausted. Although she still had some concern that her symptoms came from undetected stomach cancer, her certainty about this had dropped from 97 percent to 45 percent and her anxiety at the thought of it being cancer went from 90 percent to 30 percent.

Examining Your Evidence

Look back over your completed Worksheet 7. If you listed only one specific thought, as was the case for Joan, transfer it to the *frightening thought* column of Worksheet 8. If you listed more than one specific thought, one of them probably occurs more frequently with greater conviction or causes you more anxiety than the others. (Note that this specific thought might also be one that you listed as an overgeneralization in Worksheet 5 and may appear in the example you wrote

Worksheet 8. Collecting Evidence for and against Specific Thoughts about Health

	Evidence for the specific thought	Evidence against the specific thought
Frightening thought *Example: "The spot on my hand is skin cancer."*		
Alternative explanation *Example: "The spot on my hand is simply a freckle."*		

Source: Adapted from S. Taylor and G. J. G. Asmundson (2004). *Treating health anxiety: A cognitive-behavioral approach.* New York: Guilford Press. Adapted by permission.

	Evidence for the specific thought	Evidence against the specific thought
Frightening thought *Example: "The spot on my hand is skin cancer."* My nausea and stomach pain are from stomach cancer.	Dad had colon cancer and died from it. His symptoms were similar. He wasn't much older than me.	My symptoms are at their worst when I'm feeling overwhelmed. Unexpected things, like having to run my son to the doctor in the middle of the busy workday, bring on stomach pains. Drinking coffee and Pepsi makes things worse.
Alternative explanation *Example: "The spot on my hand is simply a freckle."* My nausea and stomach upset are from pushing myself too hard at work and not taking any time for myself.	My symptoms really flared up when my boss dumped a bunch of big projects with tight deadlines on me. Things aren't as bad when I take time out for lunch and when I eat something. Some coworkers have stomach upset and they don't have cancer. When I tried drinking less coffee and colas, like the doctor said, my heartburn went away and I started sleeping a bit better.	We have a family history of cancer.

FIGURE 4. **Joan's completed Worksheet 8.**

in Worksheet 6.) This is the specific thought you should begin working on. Transfer it to Worksheet 8. The more specific you can be in listing your thought, the more likely you'll benefit from this exercise.

Now write down any evidence to support your specific thought. Write down evidence against it. If you're stuck on coming up with an alternate explanation, think back to some of the information we presented in Chapter 2. For example, consider the following:

- Has something in your routine changed? (For Joan there was a huge increase in demands at work. Also, she'd stopped taking regular lunch breaks, wasn't eating properly, and was drinking more caffeine than usual.)
- Is your life full of stress, or has it recently become more stressful? (For Joan the added demands at work, along with minor daily hassles, were overwhelming.)
- Have you been active? (Joan was active but not exercising regularly.)
- Could you have an annoying but minor medical ailment? (Joan explored the possibility that her symptoms were the result of an ulcer. There was no medical evidence to support this possibility.)
- Is the pattern of symptoms inconsistent with what is known about the disease you fear having? (Joan learned that stomach cancer is rare in people under 50 and that it is usually associated with two symptoms—weight loss and feelings of being "full"—that she didn't have.)

If you listed more than one specific thought on Worksheet 7, you can work through this exercise for each one. The ultimate goal is to come up with an alternative explanation for your specific thoughts—a noncatastrophic, non-disease-related alternative that you believe *may* be possible. Write these alternate explanations on cards and carry them with you as a reminder to be read whenever you feel your health anxiety coming on. This is a very effective strategy for controlling your anxiety and keeping it from spiraling out of control.

Common Challenges

We sometimes see people come up with alternatives that explain their symptoms as part of a minor ailment. Joan explored this possibility in thinking that her symptoms might not be from cancer but instead from an ulcer. This is acceptable but not ideal. If you do this and if your doctor hasn't already ruled out the ailment you're considering, then have the possibility explored by your doctor. Importantly, though, try focusing on other explanations for your symptoms that aren't rooted in either major or minor sicknesses.

We've also had people ask questions such as "How can I be certain that I don't have cancer?" or comment that "Just because the tests look normal doesn't mean that I don't have multiple sclerosis. Tests can be wrong." You may have similar questions, especially if you answered *yes* to one or more of our items about all-or-none thinking. That's okay. You may find it easier to come up with non-disease-related explanations of your symptoms after working through the following simple strategy for dealing with uncertainty.

Building Emotional Muscle: Challenging Your Need for Certainty

Two things in life are certain, death and taxes. Nothing else in our lives is guaranteed. When we think about this fact, we quickly realize two things: that because we cannot avoid all risks in our lives, life is filled with uncertainty; and that all of us learn to tolerate some of the uncertainties in our lives. If you answered *yes* to one or more of the all-or-none items, you're probably having trouble accepting uncertainty about your health. If so, the following exercise will help. Using Worksheet 9, write down all of the uncertainties (about potential harm that could befall you) that you're willing to tolerate in your daily life. Spend about 10 minutes on this exercise. Be frank and honest. To help you get started, we've listed some examples of the uncertainties that we accept in our daily lives. (If some of your acceptable uncertainties are similar to ours, write them down on the worksheet.)

This exercise has several important lessons. It nicely demonstrates that you're prepared to accept all kinds of uncertainties in your life. There's no guarantee that you'll be protected from bad stuff, and yet you're prepared to accept this fact in some areas of your life. Accepting uncertainty is the only logical thing we can do and the only way we can get on with and enjoy our lives. But here's the main point of this exercise: People with health anxiety are prepared to engage in all sorts of potentially risky behaviors (for example, driving to work, eating burgers, smoking), and yet they often demand certainty when it comes to the possibility of disease. For example, Ellen, one of our patients, told us that she needed to be absolutely certain that she didn't have breast cancer. She went for test after test at the local hospital and performed breast self-exams every day, to the point that she felt sore and bruised. Although the tests were all negative, Ellen worried. "Maybe the tests have missed something." Ellen was unprepared to tolerate the possibility that there was a 0.00000001 percent chance the tests and self-exams had failed to detect cancer. As a result of her intolerance of uncertainty about breast cancer, her life was ruined; she was miserable and worried all the time.

The solution for Ellen was, first, to realize that she could accept the uncertainty (after all, she accepted all kinds of uncertainties in her life), and, second, to vigorously remind herself that she wasn't going to have her life ruined by the fact that she couldn't be absolutely certain about the medical tests. We had Ellen consider what was so bad about a little uncertainty in this area of her life and whether her need for certainty about medical tests was helping or hindering

Worksheet 9. Acceptable Uncertainties in My Life

Uncertainties that the authors of this book are prepared to accept:

- *Commuting to work, even though there's a small chance we could be killed in a car accident.*

- *Eating chicken wings, even though there's a tiny chance we could choke to death on a bone.*

- *Smoking the occasional cigar, even though nobody can guarantee that it's safe.*

- *Flying on a plane, even though it could conceivably crash.*

- *Working the occasional day at home, even though nobody can guarantee that a satellite or piece of space junk won't fall from the sky and crash through one of our roofs.*

- *Shopping in the mall, even though there's no guarantee that a crazed gunman won't kill us all.*

- *Talking on a cell phone, even though no one can give a 110 percent assurance that the electromagnetic waves from the phones are safe.*

Which uncertainties are you prepared to accept? Write them here:

her in meeting her goals in life, both at home and at work. After thinking about the matter, Ellen finally declared:

> "I owe it to myself and my family to spend my life in happy, productive ways. I'm wasting my time and ruining my quality of life by obsessing about the remote chance that I may have breast cancer. The best thing for me to do is to get the routine tests and then get on with my life."

Review your acceptable uncertainties of life as listed in Worksheet 9. If you can accept these uncertainties, don't you owe it to yourself to work on accepting some of the uncertainties that go along with medical tests and doctor visits and get on with living?

Putting Yourself in the Doctor's Shoes: Taking Another's Perspective

You might recall our suggestion that figuring out specific thoughts and worries about health and disease would be easier if you imagined how another person would view your situation or how you'd respond to a friend with the same concerns. This strategy can also be useful in changing ways of thinking that increase your health anxiety.

Has there ever been a doctor that you've admired? Perhaps your family doctor when you were a kid, or even one of the doctors on TV shows such as *ER*. Spend a few moments imagining what it would be like to be this person. Now imagine that you're the doctor and your patient is a person who has exactly the same health worries that you have. What would you, as the doctor, say to the person? Lillian, for example, awoke in the middle of the night feeling light-headed and shaky. Fearing something was seriously wrong, she woke her husband and had him drive her to the emergency room. Tests were run, and she was sent home with assurances that the symptoms were most likely due to having had a stressful day; there were no indications of physical disease on any tests. She continued waking with these symptoms on occasion, but rather than rushing to the ER, she tried thinking what the ER doctor would say to her. Taking the doctor's position, she thought:

> "You've had these symptoms before. The tests come back negative and there are no outward signs of infection or disease. We've determined that these episodes seem to occur when you push yourself too hard at work. You had a few hard days this week. Try taking it a little easier for a few days and see if this improves your sleep. It should. But, if you continue experiencing these symptoms over the next week or two, make an appointment to visit your family doctor."

This strategy worked for Lillian and helped her see that her episodes were stress related.

Try practicing this exercise using Worksheet 10. We've included a couple of examples to get you started. The purpose is to help you see your specific thoughts as assumptions that can be challenged (as in the medical detective exercise) rather than as solid facts. Breaking away from the emotions of your health anxiety will make it easier to come up with alternate explanations of what's going on in your body. It's often easier to question someone else's thoughts and worries than our own. Taking on another person's perspective allows you to do this. Some of our patients have said that this exercise is easier if they begin with less distressing thoughts. You can look back over the specific thoughts you listed on Worksheet 7 and begin this exercise with those thoughts with the lowest ratings in the "Intensity of Anxiety" column and work your way to the one with the highest rating.

Evaluating the Costs: How Bad Is It?

Many people with health anxiety jump to catastrophic conclusions about the bodily sensations they experience. The exercises described here can all be used to put these types of catastrophic misinterpretations into perspective. But some people also jump to catastrophic conclusions about the cost, or "badness," of changes in bodily sensations or of having the disease they fear. For example, one of our patients, Stan, was worried that his chronic cough, wheezing, and chest tightness meant he had chronic obstructive pulmonary disease (COPD), an incurable, noninfectious lung disease that is the fourth leading cause of death in the United States. At first he noticed the coughing and wheezing periodically throughout the day, usually early in the morning and after eating. When the wheezing became much more frequent, Stan believed that it meant two things: that the doctors were wrong and he did have COPD, and that this was going to ruin his life by rendering him completely disabled.

Several useful exercises can be used to deal with a tendency to overestimate the meaning of changes in the sensations you experience or the personal costs of disease. We had Stan answer the following questions:

- "Am I overestimating how frequent my wheezing is?"
- "Am I exaggerating how much discomfort the wheezing and coughing are causing me?"
- "Can I put up with some wheezing during the day?"
- "How bad would it be if I did have COPD or some other serious respiratory problem? Am I overestimating how bad things would be?"

After working through the questions and monitoring the frequency of symptoms (using Worksheet 1 from Chapter 2), Stan realized several things. First, his wheezing hadn't actually become more frequent. In fact, if anything, it was a little less frequent. From this he determined that he was overestimating his dis-

Worksheet 10. Putting You in the Doctor's Shoes

You as the patient	You as the doctor, responding to the patient
Write your real-life health anxieties in this column—that is, the things about your health that you really worry about these days.	Now, put on your white coat and write down the most likely cause of the patient's concerns. Remember, your mission is to make sure that your patient doesn't become needlessly worried about his or her health.
I ate beef last week. Now I'm worried about getting the human version of mad cow disease.	I ate beef, too. So did millions of people. The chances of getting sick are over a million to one. Your time on this earth is too precious for you to be worrying about rare diseases. I suggest that you spend your time on the things that give you a sense of happiness or pride; for example, pursuing fun hobbies, working on a career, or spending quality time with your friends or family.
Lately I've been feeling tired all the time. I'm frightened that I might have AIDS.	Remember that you've already had an HIV test and a number of other medical tests. The most likely causes of fatigue are stress, sleep difficulties, lack of physical fitness, boredom, and too much coffee. When you worry about feeling tired, then you might say this to yourself: "I'm very good at thinking of bad causes of tiredness, but maybe I need to think about all the harmless things that could be making me feel this way. I'll wait and see how I feel in a week or so, before consulting a doctor."
You as the patient:	You as the doctor:
You as the patient:	You as the doctor:
You as the patient:	You as the doctor:

comfort and that he could probably live with some periodic wheezing during the day. Second, he reconsidered the idea that he'd be disabled if he really did have COPD. Sure, he'd have to make some adjustments, but overall he'd do fine and, by increasing physical activity, might even wind up better off. In working through the medical-detective and building-emotional-muscle exercises, Stan realized that there was more evidence that his symptoms were related to allergy than to COPD. He became completely comfortable living with the symptoms and didn't bother going to the doctor for allergy tests.

Attention Focusing

If you answered *yes* to any of the questions in the selective-attention section, you likely focus a lot of your attention on your body, looking for bodily changes or sensations. This can lead to false alarms, wherein you believe harmless bodily noise is signaling disease. It may also explain why you seem to experience more symptoms than other people: It's not because you're sicker, it's because you focus so much attention on your body. Everyone, including healthy people, has noise in their bodies. The difference is that people with health anxiety focus more on this noise and misinterpret it as being harmful.

What do you think would happen if you focused your attention on a part of your body that you're not usually concerned about? Two areas that people don't usually focus much on include the scalp and throat. Try the following series of exercises.

- Go to a quiet room and sit in a comfortable chair. Focus on your scalp. Don't pay attention to anything else. Do this for 5 minutes. What do you notice? Do you experience any sensations that weren't there before starting? Most people notice sensations of itchiness, tingling, or tension.
- Now shift your focus to your throat. What do you notice? Many people very quickly feel a lump in the throat, feel dryness and scratchiness, and have an urge to swallow or clear their throats.
- Finally, while remaining seated, recite the alphabet in reverse order, starting from Z and working your way back to A. Do this in your head and without any movements with your hands (for example, by "writing" in the air or on the arm of your chair). Give yourself a few minutes. How did you do? Most people can't complete this task without difficulty. More important, how did your body feel during the task? Did you notice the sensations on your scalp or in your throat? Did you notice fewer sensations than usual?

We use this series of exercises to show our patients how their focus of attention has an effect on their noticing sensations in their bodies. If you focus on an area of your body, you'll notice more bodily sensations. Remember the spider demonstration from Chapter 2? Suggesting that you've seen a small spider crawling on your pant leg but aren't sure where it is now will invariably get people checking themselves and feeling itchy. People are also more likely to notice bodily sensations when bored. On the other hand, if you're keenly focused on something other than your body, you'll notice fewer bodily sensations. Joggers often listen to their favorite music as a distraction from focusing on muscle soreness. Many soldiers who are injured while absorbed in doing what they do aren't even aware that they're hurt until after the battle. The same is true of athletes engaged in their sport.

After working through this series of exercises (once or twice is usually enough for most people), you can experiment with specific bodily sensations that are related to your health worries, perhaps those you listed in Worksheet 5. Understanding how attentional focus influences your awareness of bodily sensations can help you reduce your health anxiety. It's yet another tool you have for proving you have control over your body, the sensations it produces, and whether or not they need to be responded to. As your sense of control increases, your health anxiety will decrease.

Helpful Hints and Things to Remember

We've provided you with a number of strategies for changing how and what you think about your health. Pick the strategy or combination of strategies that works best for you—the one that reduces your anxiety the most and that you're most comfortable doing—and use it consistently as a means of coping with and overcoming your anxious thoughts. Start practicing these strategies now, and continue using them in the future as you work through the other exercises in this book. You should expect to encounter a few obstacles during practice. Depending on your particular situation, these might include:

- Feeling *temporary* increases in your anxiety that prevent you from thinking clearly,
- Coming up with too few anxiety-provoking thoughts,
- Coming up with too many anxiety-provoking thoughts, and
- Having difficulty taking another person's perspective.

The good news is that these obstacles can be overcome. Try the following strategies to get back on track with your practice:

- Take a break if you feel your anxiety surging during your practice sessions. You can use the rapid relaxation or diaphragmatic breathing strategies that you learned earlier to reduce your anxiety to a point at which you're comfortable to carry on.
- If you're having difficulty coming up with anxious thoughts, try answering questions like "When I'm talking to _____ about my health concerns,

what do I say? How do I explain what I'm feeling?" and "What does _____ think about me when I'm going on about my health worries?" If this doesn't work for you, try to identify and write down your thoughts during a period when you're experiencing bodily sensation and extreme worry.

• If you come up with so many anxious thoughts you'd like to work on that you get overwhelmed and can't make any progress, try focusing your practice on just a few—no more than three—anxious thoughts. Move on to others only after you've rid yourself of these.

• If you're finding it difficult to take another person's perspective, make sure you're doing as we suggested: Start by practicing this exercise with mildly distressing thoughts and slowly work up to more distressing cognitions. With practice, you'll be successful at taking another's perspective on your most distressing thoughts and thereby form less anxiety-provoking ways of explaining it.

Over the next two weeks, you can keep track of your thoughts and the anxiety they provoke on copies of Worksheet 7. Evaluate your progress by charting the average of your daily ratings made in the "Intensity of Anxiety" column for each specific thought you have. For example, if on Friday you had three ratings, of 95, 100, and 90, for the specific worry "headache must be a brain tumor," you would tally these up and divide by 3 to get an average rating of 95. Figure 5 shows what your chart might look like. Don't be alarmed if you see small increases in anxiety ratings on some days. We often see this. What you're looking for is an overall reduction in anxiety ratings over your practice period. Even small reductions during the first two weeks of practice indicate good progress in finding alternative, non-disease-related explanations for your bodily sensations.

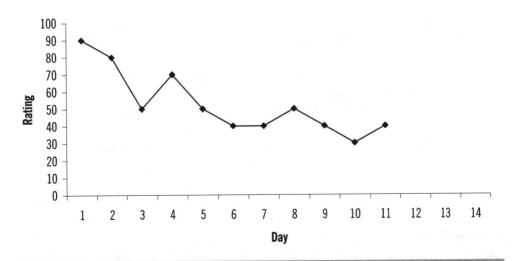

FIGURE 5. **Chart showing intensity of anxiety ratings for the specific thought that headache must be a brain tumor.**

Seven

Behaviors That Influence Your Anxiety and How to Change Them

Do you think that your health worries affect the things you do—your behavior—in any way? What sorts of things do you do to deal with your health worries? Have a quick look back at the thoughts and behaviors you wrote down on Worksheet 7 from Chapter 6 and take note of what you did to deal with your anxiety. Notice any patterns? Did you try one or more of:

- Monitoring or checking your body for changes,
- Spending time tracking down information about your signs and symptoms in books or on the Internet,
- Avoiding exercise, leisure activities you once enjoyed, or spending time with your family and friends,
- Taking medications or having a medical procedure that wasn't recommended,
- Trying to get a family member or friend to tell you everything was okay, or
- Thinking about visiting your doctor?

These are a few common examples. There are, in fact, many different, well-intentioned things that people with health anxiety do to cope with their worries. Sarah, whom you met in Chapter 1, was repeatedly visiting her doctor to see if her breast lumps were cancerous. She was also checking her breasts for changes with great frequency, at least once per hour every day. Bob, also from

Chapter 1, was avoiding public washrooms and other public situations because he feared catching an infectious disease. Because complete avoidance wasn't possible, he started wearing latex gloves and developed his "foot technique" for opening doors, lifting toilet seats, and flushing. Matt, one of our patients discussed later in this chapter, spent hours searching the Internet for information about the signs and symptoms of chest pain.

How you behave when you're anxious about your health is important because, although worries that you have a serious disease or are at risk of catching one can influence your behavior, the reverse is also true. Your behavior can influence the amount of health anxiety you feel—some behaviors keep your anxiety alive, whereas others reduce it. In the first part of this chapter we'll focus on behaviors that feed the health anxiety cycle. These fall into four main groups as follows:

1. Repetitive checking for body changes and sensations or of health information sources,
2. Avoiding things that increase health anxiety,
3. Seeking reassurance from doctors, family, and friends that everything is okay, and
4. Relying on things that are emotionally comforting or believed to be linked to the absence of disease.

You need to understand these behaviors and how they affect you if you're going to conquer your health anxiety. This will be the focus of week 11 of our program. In the second part of the chapter, we'll build on this understanding by teaching you some simple strategies for changing your anxiety-maintaining behaviors and replacing them with ways of doing things that will increase your sense of well-being (weeks 12 through 14). If you've been practicing the exercises from Chapter 5, you'll already have a head start on this by having become better at managing the stress in your life.

Identifying Behaviors That Feed Health Anxiety: Week 11

Repetitive Checking

If you've ever baked cookies or roasted a chicken, you've probably peeked into the oven several times to see if they were ready. A few people we know double-check that they've locked their car doors or have their keys in hand before leaving the parking lot. One of our wives sometimes checks her departure time and gate a few times while waiting for a connecting flight. And each day one of us checks his e-mail several times (actually, too many times) to make sure he doesn't miss any urgent messages. We're all told by our doctors that we should be doing regular breast or testicular self-examinations. The bottom line is that when concerned about something, most people will check and sometimes recheck to make sure things are going the way they should. It's human nature to do so.

Some checking, as in the previous examples, seems to be useful; it prevents burnt food, leaving the car unlocked, and overlooking early signs of cancer. It doesn't interfere with our daily activities. But some people with obsessive–compulsive disorder spend a great amount of time checking things. One of our patients, for example, felt compelled to go through an elaborate ritual every night before going to bed. He'd repeatedly check that all of the electrical appliances in his house were unplugged, that the stove was correctly turned off, and that the doors and windows were locked. Some nights it would take him over an hour to complete his checking ritual. People with health anxiety often spend a lot of time checking their bodies. Some also spend a lot of time checking for and reading information on disease.

Body Checking

Because we've already talked about body checking in Chapter 2, we won't spend a lot of time on it here. But one key piece of information is important to keep in mind: Focusing attention on something increases the chances of its being noticed. What happens when a mother listens carefully for sounds from the baby after putting her newborn to bed? What about a young teenager who's spending a whole night all alone at home for the first time? They hear almost every single noise in the house. The same is true when we turn our attention inward on the functioning of our bodies. We notice bodily noises that we might have otherwise overlooked; noises typical of the functioning of a healthy body. You're more likely to have a false alarm—to think this noise means you're sick—if you have beliefs (or specific thoughts) that certain bodily sensations are symptoms of disease and if you have an amplifying somatic style (that is, if you scored high on the Whiteley Index from Chapter 1). The attention-focusing strategies that you learned in Chapter 6 can help with this. We'll teach you some other strategies for dealing with body checking later in this chapter.

Checking Health Information

Some people with health anxiety spend a lot of time searching for information about diseases. Books, magazines, and TV shows about disease are common sources of this information. Some people with health anxiety repeatedly call health information hotlines. For example, they may call hotlines set up for general health concerns, such as fever, or more specific diseases, such as AIDS. But, by far, the most frequently used source for learning about signs and symptoms of disease is the Internet. It has put a wealth of medical information and misinformation at our fingertips.

What purpose do you think checking information on health and disease serves? Our patients usually give one of two answers to this question. First, they say they want to find information that shows that their bodily sensations or changes are in fact harmless. They hope to learn that everything is okay. Second, they say they want to learn ways of preventing diseases. For example, they want to know which foods to eat and which to avoid to keep from getting cancer or how to best kill kitchen bacteria after cooking.

These are admirable goals. Indeed, they're very similar to some of the things cognitive-behavioral therapists hope their patients will do. They're also in line with what we want you to get from working through this book—more knowledge about how your body works and how to live life to its fullest. Unfortunately, when people with health anxiety search for information, they usually turn up "facts" that are more alarming than they are helpful. This feeds their health anxiety cycle and often makes things worse. There are a couple of reasons for this.

As we've discussed before, people with health anxiety sometimes catastrophically misinterpret the information they find. For example, after reading a magazine article, Jackson became interested in learning the best way of cleaning his kitchen to reduce germs. He found several Internet sites that suggested he'd been improperly cleaning his kitchen after handling chicken. They also indicated that the way he was now cleaning up was putting him and his family at risk of getting food poisoning and possibly dying from it. He became so alarmed that he stopped buying chicken (a family favorite), wouldn't let anyone else cook, was spending a lot of time cleaning the kitchen after every meal, and began searching for other information about food-related bacteria and diseases. Did Jackson overreact? His goal of killing bacteria was a good one. But his worries about contamination and death from the bacteria were exaggerated and, unfortunately, caused problems with his wife and kids (who wanted to eat chicken and spend time with him after supper).

Whenever Matt experienced chest pain, he'd go to the Internet and search medical websites for information. His cardiologist had told him his heart was healthy and that his pains were caused by stress-related muscle tension. He hoped to find information that would confirm this. Instead, he found information indicating that chest pain like his was a symptom of several heart conditions, some rare and deadly. He also saw a news report indicating that he was at particularly high risk for these conditions, given his age, weight, and ethnicity. He became so worried about dying from heart failure that he insisted his cardiologist perform a series of very risky tests to rule out these rare diseases. The tests all indicated that he had a healthy heart.

Although people seek them out as a source of good information, many newspaper articles, newsletters, magazines, and TV news reports and shows on disease contain inaccurate information. This was the case with the news report

Matt saw. Others are purposefully exaggerated or sensationalized for impact. Inaccurate and exaggerated claims aren't easy to identify when they come from a trusted source. Take, for example, the following quote from a widely read health newsletter:

> Germs that can make you sick are everywhere. According to an unpublished University of Arizona study, playground equipment, handrails and armrests, surfaces in public bathrooms, and shopping cart handles are among the *surfaces* that are likely to have traces of saliva or other bodily fluids that could contain germs. The *places* where you've got to be especially careful: daycare centers, gyms, doctors' offices, and restaurants. . . . And cold bugs can survive on your skin for several hours. So if you rub your eyes or scratch your nose—the main routes of entry—after touching a contaminated surface, the germs can hitch a ride right into your body. (*Nutrition Action Healthletter*, March 2002)

The suggestion that we're all at imminent risk of being contaminated by germs if we leave our homes, whether out of necessity (to take our kids to day care) or pleasure (for a nice meal), is exaggerated. The effect of inaccurate and exaggerated information on health anxiety is similar to the effect of catastrophic misinterpretations: It increases health anxiety and further fuels that need to get more information. Many of the strategies that you learned about in Chapters 5 and 6, as well as some that we discuss later in this chapter, are helpful in reducing the urge to check health-related information.

Avoidance

Our bodies are designed in a way that increases the likelihood that we'll survive threats to our well-being. The "fight or flight" response—activated by the sympathetic division of our autonomic nervous system—helps us fight back or get away from things that might be dangerous to us. Most people try to avoid things that are uncomfortable, painful, or fear provoking. Avoidance is also a common response of people with health anxiety when they have to deal with people, things, or activities related in some way to their health worries. There are several ways of avoiding things, and the specific pattern of avoidance can depend on the type of health anxiety you have.

If you worry that you have a particular disease, you've probably *stopped doing things* that you think will make your condition worse. Matt, for example, avoided biking, hiking, and playing with his children—activities he had once enjoyed—for fear that too much physical activity would increase the strain on his heart and cause it to stop beating. Gertrude was so worried that she had lung cancer that she avoided leaving the house whenever possible so that she didn't come into contact with secondhand smoke. She also stopped exercising because she didn't like feeling breathless and didn't want to overstress her lungs. Matt and

Gertrude were avoiding two things—certain activities and bodily sensations caused by the activities.

You might also have *started doing things* to avoid a feared outcome, such as dying. Wanting to avoid a heart attack, Lachlan bought his own machine for checking his blood pressure. He checked it about six times a day. The type of avoidance characterized by not doing things is called *passive avoidance*; the type in which you start doing things is called *active avoidance*.

People who are afraid of catching a disease usually have a passive avoidance style. They avoid doing things that they think will increase their risk of actually catching something. Bob did whatever he could (and was quite creative in doing so) to avoid skin contact with any part of public washrooms used. Mike, who feared catching SARS, wouldn't allow his friend from Toronto to come for a visit. He stopped having other company as well, thinking that they could have visited Toronto or some other high-risk area without his knowing. Gina stopped visiting her family and friends who had pets because she was afraid of getting rabies. She'd also given up jogging in the park and volunteering at the animal shelter, two activities she once loved.

What are the consequences of trying to cope by using avoidance? What does the person who is doing the avoiding get out of it? Are there benefits? Are there drawbacks? There are, in fact, both benefits and drawbacks. The benefit of avoidance is that you don't have to experience the bodily sensation, activity, or thing that makes you uncomfortable or of which you're afraid. Being able to stay away from these things brings about a feeling of relief. It's for this reason that many people with health anxiety develop a habit of coping by avoiding. The unfortunate truth is that the relief provided by avoidance is short-lived. Anxiety soon returns. Why? As we mentioned in Chapter 5, you need to confront the things that make you anxious to triumph over anxiety! One of us has a daughter who loves to swim and play about in the water. She wasn't always that way. When she was taken to her first swimming lesson she was terrified. She expressed worries and dislike for the water on the way to a large number of her lessons. One week we couldn't make it to the lesson because of a snowstorm, and she was relieved; overjoyed, in fact! Wanting her to learn to swim, we worked on her discomfort (by pointing out how great it'd be to be able to swim at the lake and with friends) and persisted in taking her to lessons. It was only by taking her to the pool over and over again and by showing her that she was safe in the water that we helped her to overcome her anxieties. Later in this chapter, we'll show you how your avoidance of things that you've come to associate with your health anxiety can be overcome in much the same way.

Reassurance Seeking

People with health anxiety, such as Matt, often seek out information on disease because they hope they'll learn that everything is okay. Like Sarah, introduced in Chapter 1, Matt was also visiting his doctor on a monthly basis to discuss his symptoms and make sure he wasn't sick. *Reassurance seeking* is a term we use to describe the behavior of getting information, usually from doctors, that signs and symptoms aren't related to disease. Reassurance can be thought of as the repeated presentation of the simple message that there's nothing physically wrong and that there's no evidence of disease.

The benefits and drawbacks of reassurance seeking are much the same as those of avoidance. The benefit is an almost immediate feeling of relief and reduced anxiety. Research has shown that this occurs, but it also shows that the feelings of relief don't last long. Health anxiety usually returns within 24 hours, often when bodily sensations or changes are noticed again. This leads to questions such as "Why would I be experiencing more symptoms if my doctor said I was healthy?" and "I wonder if the doctor missed something or if the tests were faulty." These questions increase health anxiety for those who don't like uncertainty, and the result is more information seeking—more reading, more surfing the Internet, more doctor visits, and more medical tests. This feeds the health anxiety cycle by keeping attention focused on bodily sensations and changes and by increasing the chances of finding alarming information. By relying on doctors to placate worries, the health-anxious person doesn't get an opportunity to learn that the feared bodily sensations are harmless. He or she doesn't take that all-important step of testing the waters on his or her own.

Security Blankets

The *Peanuts* comic strip created by Charles M. Schulz, featuring Charlie Brown and his friends, is one of the most successful and enduring cartoons of our time. One of Charlie Brown's friends, Linus Van Pelt, inspired the term *security blanket* with his unwillingness to go anywhere or do anything without his favorite baby-blue comforter. Like Linus, we all have security blankets of one sort or another—things that are emotionally comforting and that make us feel safe. For some it's a tub of chocolate ice cream. For others it may be a warm bath or a favorite pair of pajamas. For people with health anxiety it's *anything* that's believed to give protection from disease or medical emergency. The list of possible security blankets is almost endless, but here are some examples:

- Wearing a MedicAlert bracelet,
- Wearing latex gloves,
- Carrying a cellular phone,
- Carrying bottles of prescription medication,
- Keeping a doctor's business card handy in a purse or wallet,
- Purchasing medical testing equipment, such as blood pressure monitors or cardiac defibrillators, for personal use, and
- Living close to a hospital.

In each case, the security blanket provides the person with a sense of safety from possible threats to his or her health.

The use of security blankets seems harmless. But relying on them for relief from health-related worries feeds the health anxiety cycle. Why might this be? First, although they provide some comfort, the security blankets are also reminders of disease. Matt carried nitroglycerin pills around in his pocket. He found comfort in knowing the pills would keep his heart pumping if it began beating too slowly. The pills were also a constant reminder of the fear that his heart would stop beating. This reminder fed his specific thoughts about the various rare heart conditions he might have and made him worry more. Second, reliance on security blankets as a way of coping keeps people feeling helpless and unable to take control over their situations. They feel uncomfortable and unable to do anything without their security blankets. To break the health anxiety cycle, it's necessary to give up security blankets.

Things to Remember

People with health anxiety do many different things to cope with their worries. These things usually fit into one of four groups—repetitive checking, avoidance, reassurance seeking, and reliance on security blankets. By looking over the things you wrote down in the last column on Worksheet 7 from Chapter 6, you'll get an idea of the things you do to deal with your health anxiety. We'll also give you some exercises in the next section to get a better handle on this. The things you're doing are most likely providing you some relief from anxiety. But the relief they provide is always going to be short-lived, and your anxiety will return. If this weren't the case, you wouldn't be reading this book. A question we're often asked is "Why do people keep using these ways of coping if they don't work all that well?" The answer is that it's the temporary relief from anxiety that keeps people using them. Our goal for this chapter is to teach you strategies that will give you more than temporary relief.

Getting Rid of Behaviors That Feed Health Anxiety: Weeks 12 to 14

The next step in conquering your health anxiety is to get rid of any anxiety-feeding behaviors you have. These will be replaced with behaviors that give you a greater sense of control over your well-being. We're going to show you several different strategies for doing this. These include:

- Testing the effectiveness of checking and reassurance seeking,
- Confronting feared bodily sensations and feared situations, and
- Letting go of security blankets.

We recommend that you work through the steps provided for each of these strategies *before* starting to practice any of them. You can then pick the ones that seem best matched to you—the ones you think will help you get rid of the specific things you're doing to feed your health anxiety—and practice those. Focused practice should last at least three weeks, although in some cases it may take a little longer. You can expect to add a few weeks of practice if you're working on more than one strategy for replacing your health anxiety behaviors. We've mentioned a few times that an important part of these exercises is coming face-to-face with the things that you're afraid of. Have we convinced you that confronting the things you fear is the best way to overcome them? If not, ask yourself the following question: "Have the things I've been doing to this point— things like checking the Internet, seeing my doctor, and avoiding things I really want to do—helped me conquer my anxiety?" The answer will probably be no. We like to think of our exercises as an investment of a little short-term pain for a big long-term gain. You're already experiencing long-term pain from your health anxiety, so what do you have to lose?

Several of the strategies in this chapter are designed to *gradually* expose you to the things you fear. This gradual approach will allow you to get used to your feelings before moving on. So, once you've decided to work on a particular strategy, practice the exercises in the order we present them. Don't skip ahead! Most of what you'll feel—increased heart rate, shortness of breath, light-headedness, and shakiness—is related to your body's stress reaction. Don't fight the stress reaction. Let it happen. Some people may also feel a bit irritable or develop a headache. Don't be alarmed by these feelings. They're not dangerous, and they'll pass within a short time. Instead, we encourage you to think of your stress reaction, increased anxiousness, and other feelings that go along with it as evidence that you're actually working on the right exercises for you. Although it sounds a little silly, it's true that the exercises that make you feel anxious are the same ones that will help break your health anxiety cycle.

Testing the Effectiveness of Checking and Reassurance Seeking

Checking and reassurance seeking feed the health anxiety cycle in slightly different ways, but the exercises that will help you to give them up are almost identical. We'll teach you to test the effectiveness of these behaviors as a way of coping using a step-by-step approach. Our goal is to have you learn for yourself that these behaviors aren't helpful in the long term. Ultimately, we want you to give up checking and reassurance seeking almost completely.

Step 1: Identify Your Checking and Reassurance-Seeking Behaviors

Using Worksheet 11, list all of the checking behaviors that you remember doing. You may have only one, or you may have several. Some of these behaviors may

Worksheet 11.
My Checking and Reassurance-Seeking Behaviors

Type	What I do
Bodily checking	
Searching for information	
Reassurance seeking	

be obvious to you—for example, repeatedly checking for bodily sensations or changes, searching for medical information on the Internet, and visiting your doctor for reassurance. Others, such as telling your family or friends about your symptoms in hopes that they'll tell you everything is okay, may not be as obvious. You can add to the list whenever something comes to mind. An example of Matt's partially completed Worksheet 11 is shown in Figure 6.

Type	What I do
Bodily checking	• *I pay close attention to my heart and the way it beats.* • *I take my pulse at least 10 times a day. I count beats for a few minutes and try to feel times when the pause between them is longer than usual.*
Searching for information	• *I spend most of my free time surfing the Internet for information about chest pain and types of heart disease. About 3 hours or more each day.* • *When not on the Internet I try to watch programs about heart disease and its effects. I sometimes tape them and watch them late at night.*
Reassurance seeking	• *I go to my family doctor at least once a month to make sure I'm not going to drop dead. Have done this for past year or so.* • *I've seen a cardiologist a few times recently for the same reason.*

FIGURE 6. **Matt's checking and reassurance-seeking behaviors.**

Step 2: Identify Advantages and Disadvantages

Revisiting a strategy you've already learned, examine the evidence for the advantages and disadvantages of the behaviors you identified in Step 1. Make a copy of Worksheet 12 for each of your checking and reassurance-seeking behaviors and write down the advantages and disadvantages of each. By having read the earlier parts of this book, you've already gathered most of the information you'll need to do this. Also, try to come up with an alternative behavior that you might replace your checking behavior with. Write down its advantages and disadvantages, as well. Consider, for example, what would happen if you stopped doing what you're doing; or what might happen if you started doing the behavior *more often* over a period of a week or so. You may find it odd that we'd ask you to do more of something that feeds your health anxiety. But we often ask our patients to do this because doing more of something is a good way of showing exactly how it affects health anxiety. Take a few minutes to work through this step now. An example of Matt's completed Worksheet 12 for surfing the Internet for medical information is shown in Figure 7. Use it as a guide to get yourself started.

Do the disadvantages you listed for your checking or reassurance-seeking behaviors outweigh the advantages? If you answered *yes*, you're ready to begin work on giving up these behaviors and replacing them with alternative ones. Step 3 will help you do this. If you answered *no*, then carefully review the first section of this chapter, as well as Chapters 1 and 2, and see if this helps you find some more disadvantages. If it does, move on to Step 3. If not, you can still move on to Step 3. You may find it a little more challenging to work through, but if you stick to it, the results will come.

Step 3: Practice Alternative Behaviors

Take a look at Table 5. It shows some examples of sample exercises and what will be learned from each. As with the alternative behaviors you identified in Step 2, the sample exercises fall into categories of decreasing or increasing a behavior. How do the sample exercises compare with the alternative behaviors you wrote down for yourself on Worksheet 12? People with health anxiety have many different ways of checking and seeking reassurance. Over the next week we want you to practice the alternative behaviors you came up with. If you stick to it, what you'll see for yourself is that:

- Increasing your checking behavior makes things worse,
- Decreasing it doesn't cause a health catastrophe, and
- Doing these exercises repeatedly leads to a decrease in your health anxiety.

Worksheet 12.
Collecting Evidence of Advantages and Disadvantages
of My Checking and Reassurance Seeking Behaviors

	Advantages	Disadvantages
Behavior *Example: "I check the mole on my arm throughout the day, poking and picking at it to see if it's changed color or grown."*		
Alternative behavior *Example: "I could stop checking the mole" or "I could start checking more often, say every two hours for the next four days."*		

	Advantages	**Disadvantages**
Behavior *Example: "I check the mole on my arm throughout the day, poking and picking at it to see if it's changed color or grown."* I spend most of my free time surfing the Internet for information about chest pain and heart disease.	• I'll know whatever there is to know about the causes of chest pain. • I'll know everything I need to know about heart disease and how to keep myself from dropping dead. • If there are any new discoveries I'll know about them right away.	• I don't have time to do anything else and really have no interest in anything else. It's always worrying about my heart stopping. • I'm falling behind at work because I keep sneaking on the Internet. • I feel really bad about not spending time with my wife and kids. I get frustrated when they interrupt my Internet time, and then I feel bad about this. I think they're fed up with me.
Alternative behavior *Example: "I could stop checking the mole" or "I could start checking more often, say every two hours for the next four days."* I could stop surfing the Internet. That's my goal. But first I'm going to see what happens if I spend as much time searching for information as I can.	• Asmundson and Taylor say that I'll learn for myself that surfing is keeping my health anxiety alive. If I can kick this habit then maybe I can start spending some good quality time with my family. • Maybe I'll also be able to dig out from under the mountain of work I've let pile up.	• If I stop surfing I could miss some important medical breakthrough that could benefit me. • Spending more time on the Internet can't make things much worse than they already are. I'm on almost all of the time.

FIGURE 7. **Matt's advantages and disadvantages of checking the Internet for medical information.**

TABLE 5. **Sample Exercises and Learning Objectives for Testing the Effectiveness of Checking and Reassurance-Seeking Behaviors**

Behavior	Sample exercise	Learning objective
Body checking—lymph nodes	Repeatedly check lymph nodes by repeated palpation (versus not checking)	Repeated checking is a cause of bodily swelling and tenderness
Body checking—lump in throat	Checking throat by repeatedly swallowing (versus not swallowing)	A feared sensation (lump in the throat) is caused by repeated swallowing
Information checking—surfing the Internet	Refrain, for one week, from looking up medical information on the Internet or in books	Refraining from collecting medical information has no adverse impact on my health
Going to the doctor for medical reassurance	Seeking medical reassurance weekly versus putting it off for a month	Reassurance seeking feeds my preoccupation with health and disease
Talking with family members for reassurance	Ask family to refrain from giving reassurance	My preoccupation with health and disease declines when reassurance is not given

Source: Adapted from S. Taylor and G. J. G. Asmundson (2004). *Treating health anxiety: A cognitive-behavioral approach.* New York: Guilford Press. Adapted by permission.

    This was exactly the case for Matt. He decided to try spending five days doing almost nothing but surfing the Internet in his spare time. This was followed by five days without surfing at all. He monitored his activities and anxiety levels. Worksheet 13 can be used to assist you in monitoring your behavioral exercises. Matt also kept track of his specific thoughts using Worksheet 7 from Chapter 6. What he found was that his anxiety about his heart stopping was high when surfing and gradually became lower during the days he wasn't surfing. Related to this, he noticed having fewer specific thoughts about his heart malfunctioning when not surfing. He learned that surfing the Internet was making his health anxiety worse rather than better.

Helpful Hints

Our purpose in asking you to test the effectiveness of checking and reassurance-seeking behaviors is for you to learn that nothing bad will happen if you give them up and to recognize for yourself that doing so will reduce your feelings of anxiety. We pretty much want you to give up these behaviors completely. But *completely* may be asking a lot. Some people can do this. Others can for a while but then lapse and start checking or seeking reassurance again. If this happens to

Worksheet 13. Monitoring Form for Behavioral Exercises.

Day and date	Exercise	Peak anxiety (0–100)	What did you learn from the exercise?
Example 1	Spent 5 min feeling the lymph glands on neck, to see if they were swollen	50	Repeated checking and squeezing makes my glands feel sore and swollen. Repeated checking creates problems— it makes me think my glands are swollen.
Example 2	Jogged around the block	70	I was worried that my body couldn't take the exertion. But I survived! Maybe I'm not as frail as I thought.
Example 3	Walked past a funeral home	65	Nothing bad happened. I can't get sick by being near dead bodies.

Source: From S. Taylor and G. J. G. Asmundson (2004). Treating health anxiety: A cognitive-behavioral approach. New York: Guilford Press. Reprinted by permission.

you, don't despair. Instead, you can turn your lapse into a learning experience. Work through the steps of this exercise again from the beginning. Sometimes it's necessary to show yourself all over again that your alternatives to checking and reassurance seeking decrease your anxiety in the long run.

Keep in mind that some checking behaviors are good for us when done in moderation. If you're repeatedly checking for lumps in your breasts or testicles, we don't want you to stop completely. Instead, set up a schedule to do a self-exam once a month. Mark a date on your calendar and do the self-exam only when the date arrives. If you have a strong urge to start checking your body or looking for medical information, remember that turning your attention to something else will help. If you busy yourself with another task, the urge will pass.

Also keep in mind that seeing your family doctor for annual physical examinations is important. Scheduling your annual exams ahead of time and marking them on your calendar is a useful way of keeping track of but not overfocusing your attention on the appointment date. If symptoms arise before your annual exam, they may or may not need medical attention. That is, they may or may not be due to anxiety. You may want to give in and seek reassurance from your doctor that you're not sick. In this case, we strongly recommend a wait-and-see approach. If the symptoms persist for more than a week despite your working through the other strategies you've learned in this book—stress management and changing anxiety-provoking thoughts—then and only then go to the doctor.

Confronting Feared Bodily Sensations and Situations

Cognitive-behavioral therapists like to use exercises called *exposure* to help people get over their fears. Exposure is a strategy designed to get you to come face-to-face with the things you fear and feel anxious about. Because many people with health anxiety are afraid of bodily sensations and changes, we're going to ask you to work through exercises in which you'll purposefully bring on these sensations or changes in your body. These exercises, called *interoceptive exposure*, are designed to give you extra evidence that your bodily sensations and changes aren't a sign that you're sick and that, in fact, they are very much under your control. The exercises for confronting feared situations, called *situational exposure*, are very similar to those for confronting feared bodily sensations. You'll want to try these exercises if you avoid certain things, people, or places that you fear will make your condition worse. The goal of situational exposure is to provide evidence that doing certain things you've associated with disease doesn't really put you at a higher risk for developing the disease.

Not everybody needs to practice both types of exposure. Some people are more worried about bodily sensations and changes, whereas others worry more about doing certain things. If your biggest worries are about bodily sensations or changes, then interoceptive exposure will likely be best for you. On the other hand, situational exposure might work best if you worry more about doing things or even avoid doing them because they make you anxious. We'll explain the steps for each type of exposure and let you decide whether to do one or both. The steps for doing interoceptive and situational exposure are similar and include:

- Identifying the specific things that make you most anxious,
- Choosing the best exposure exercise for you, and
- Practicing your exposure exercises.

Interoceptive Exposure

Step 1: Identify the Sensations and Changes That Make You Most Anxious. Choosing the interoceptive exposure exercises you'll do depends on which bodily sensations and changes make you feel most anxious. Is it a racing heart, shortness of breath, headache, fatigue, muscle pain, stomach cramps, light-headedness, shakiness, hot flashes, seeing "stars" floating in front of your eyes, skin rash, lumps under the skin, moles, or something else along these lines? Reviewing your worksheets from Chapters 2 and 6 will help you pinpoint the ones you're most worried about. Write them on the following lines. If you worry a lot about more than three bodily sensations or changes, write down the three that cause you the most worry. These are the ones you'll work on. Using our 0-to-100 scale, with 0 being *no anxiety* and 100 being *extreme anxiety*, make a note of how anxious these sensations or changes make you feel right now.

1. _____
2. _____
3. _____

Step 2: Choose the Best Exposure Exercise for You. Table 6 shows examples of some interoceptive exposure exercises that can be performed for various bodily sensations and changes. For example, if you worry that heart palpitations mean you're going to have a heart attack, you could try fast-paced running on the spot for two minutes. Or you might go to a 30-minute aerobics class. The purpose of these exercises is to show how certain activities bring on a rapid heart rate and that this rapid heart rate is a normal bodily response. It's important for you to know that everyone can do exposure exercises but that not all exposure exercises are for everyone. In other words, certain exercises shouldn't be done in some cases. If you have a medical condition that's been *confirmed* by your doctor, caution may be needed. There are some exercises that you shouldn't do. For instance, a person with asthma shouldn't do exercises involving hyperventilation

TABLE 6. **Examples of Interoceptive Exposure Exercises**

Exercise	Learning objective: The following sensations have no harmful consequences
Hyperventilate, taking a deep breath in and out every second, for 1 minute	Dizziness, dry mouth, breathlessness, racing heart, tingling, trembling or shakiness
Shake your head side to side for 30 seconds	Dizziness, light-headedness
Place your head between knees for 30 seconds and then rapidly sit upright	Light-headedness
Breathe through a narrow straw for 2 minutes	Shortness of breath, smothering feelings, dizziness, light-headedness, chest tightness, trembling or shakiness
Exhale and then hold your breath for 30 seconds	Chest tightness, shortness of breath, light-headedness, racing heart
Breathe with chest muscles rather than diaphragm	Chest tightness
Swallow and then hold your throat in "mid-swallow" for 10 seconds	Throat tightness, lump in throat
Swallow five times in a row very quickly	Throat tightness, lump in throat
Clear your throat five times quickly	Sore throat
Carry a heavy bag of groceries for 60 seconds	Trembling or shakiness, breathlessness, racing or pounding heart, light-headedness, muscle tension and fatigue
Drink hot coffee	Racing heart, sweating, hot flashes
Sit in a chair and then tense all of your muscles for 1 minute	Muscle tension, trembling or shakiness, light-headedness
Jog on the spot or run up and down stairs for 2 minutes	Racing heart, chest tightness, breathlessness, smothering feelings, sweating, hot flashes, muscle tension and fatigue
Do a 30-minute aerobics class	Racing heart, chest tightness, breathlessness, fatigue, sweating, muscle tension and fatigue

Source: Adapted from S. Taylor and G. J. G. Asmundson (2004). *Treating health anxiety: A cognitive-behavioral approach.* New York: Guilford Press. Adapted by permission.

to bring on dizziness, and a person with migraine headaches may be better off not drinking caffeinated beverages to promote sweating. If you do have a confirmed medical condition and you are unsure whether you should do a particular exposure exercise, discuss your concerns with your doctor. The doctor will tell you whether the exercise is something you can do.

There are several ways to decide which exercises to do. First, you can select exercises from Table 6 that match up with your feared bodily sensations or changes. Second, you can try exposing yourself to behaviors that you've been avoiding to keep from experiencing certain bodily sensations—for example, walking up the stairs if you fear heart palpitations. Finally, you can use a combination of these two methods. Whatever exercises you choose to do, you should start with ones that you're fairly confident you'll be able to do for the duration of the exercise. Write down the exercises that you think will work for you on the following lines. Now, using another 0-to-100 scale, with 0 equal to *not at all confident* and 100 equal to *completely confident,* rate your confidence in fully doing each exercise you've selected. Most of our patients list at least one exercise that they're fairly certain they can complete.

1. _____
2. _____
3. _____

Start by practicing the exercises that you rated close to 70. By doing this you'll ensure starting out with manageable exercises—something that's challenging but not impossible—and you'll slowly build confidence in taking on the challenge of more distressing exercises. Matt used a combination of the first and second methods to select his exposure exercises. He started daily jogging on the spot for two minutes, something he had 85 percent confidence in being able to do. He did this for a week. As his confidence grew, he added biking every second day for 20 minutes over the next week and then daily roughhousing with his kids. At first he didn't have much confidence in being able to get through these last two tasks, with initial ratings of 55 percent and 40 percent, but as he worked his way through the jogging exercise his confidence increased to a point that he felt okay about giving them a try.

Step 3: Practice Your Exposure Exercises. All interoceptive exposure exercises are meant to be brief and should take only a few minutes each. We recommend that you practice each exercise selected in Step 2 several times a day. The more you practice these exercises, gradually exposing yourself to feared bodily sensations, the less distressing they'll become. Add exercises as your confidence in being able to work through them increases to above 70. For any given exercise this could take anywhere from a few days to a few weeks.

Situational Exposure

Step 1: Identify Things That Make You Most Anxious. Exercise and other physical activities are often avoided because they cause bodily sensations associated with an impending health crisis of some sort, such as heart attack or ruptured aneurysm. Gradually adding these activities to your interoceptive exposure exercises will reduce the anxiety they cause and, if you stick with it, will also improve your physical fitness. You can try exposing yourself to different kinds of activities and monitor how they make you feel using the steps outlined here. Because almost anything can be linked to a disease in some way or other, people with disease phobia avoid an endless number of situations because of fear of catching a disease. Some examples include avoiding visiting people in hospitals, reading or watching shows about sick people, going to parties or restaurants where smoking is allowed, touching public doors, using public washrooms, and so on. Reviewing the worksheets from Chapter 6 may help you pinpoint the situations you're most worried about. Write down the three that cause you the most worry on the following lines. Using our 0-to-100 scale, with 0 being *no anxiety* and 100 being *extreme anxiety*, make a note of how anxious these situations would make you feel if you were in them.

1. _____
2. _____
3. _____

Step 2: Choose the Best Exposure Exercise for You. Table 7 shows examples of things that can be used in situational exposure exercises to overcome fear of catching various diseases. You can select from these examples and use them as a guide for making up exercises that are specific to the things you avoid. To do this you'll need to think about the many different things related to the diseases you're afraid of catching.

• Using Worksheet 14, write down everything you can think of that's related to your top-ranked situations. Write down as many things as you can, without judging whether you think they're possible to do and without rating how anxious they'd make you feel if you did them. Try to get down at least 10 different things.

• Cross out anything you wrote down that wouldn't be possible to do. For example, if you wrote down "visit a cancer ward" or "walk through a 'rough' part of town" but live in a place that doesn't have these things, you'd cross them off your list.

• Using the 0–100 scale, rate how much anxiety you'd feel if you were actually in each situation that hasn't been crossed out. If the same or a very similar

TABLE 7. **Examples of Things That Can Be Used in Situational Exposure Exercises for Some Commonly Feared Diseases**

Fear of contracting . . .	Items and activities that can be used for exposure exercises
Cancer	• Magazine photos of people who battled cancer • Illustrated textbooks on cancer • TV documentaries on cancer • Hospital cancer wards
Airborne germs	• Walking past funeral homes • Sitting in a hospital waiting room where sick people have been sitting • The sight and sound of a person coughing (e.g., the therapist) • Talking to people who appear to be ill
HIV	• Illustrated articles on HIV • TV programs on HIV • Walking in a "gay" part of town • Volunteering at a hospice for HIV-positive people
Food poisoning	• Eating tinned foods without washing the tins beforehand • Eating unusual or unfamiliar foods (e.g., exotic fruits that have been washed before consumption) • Cooking and eating chicken that is one day past the "use by" date • Dining in a "cheap-looking" cafe
Rabies	• Visiting a pet store and handling puppies • Walking in a park frequented by people walking their dogs • Looking at dogs in a local pound • Volunteering as a dog-walker at a pound

Source: From S. Taylor and G. J. G. Asmundson (2004). *Treating health anxiety: A cognitive-behavioral approach*. New York: Guilford Press. Reprinted by permission.

rating was given to more than one activity, choose the one that you want to try doing and cross out the others.

• Cross out any remaining activities that aren't really related or that don't fit well with the others. Your goal is to get down to around four to seven activities, with anxiety ratings ranging from low to high.

• Copy your list on a separate piece of paper so that it goes from the activity that you rated as causing the least anxiety to the one rated as causing the most anxiety. This is your situational exposure exercise list for your top-ranked situation. A completed example of Worksheet 14 is shown in Figure 8.

Again, baby steps are important. If you start by practicing the exercises that you rated as least anxiety provoking, you'll slowly build confidence to work through the ones you rated as more distressing. Francis, for example, avoided going anywhere near hospitals because he feared contracting a serious disease

Worksheet 14.
Things Related to Situations I'm Afraid of

Situation: _____

Situation: _I avoid being anywhere near sick people_

Drive past a hospital   35

Walk past a hospital   53

~~Watch ER   40~~   (doesn't fit with other activities)

~~Read articles about contagious diseases   45~~   (doesn't fit with other activities)

~~Visit a friend whose kids have a cold   90~~   (no friends have a cold right now)

Walk through a hospital parking lot   64

Walk up to a hospital entrance   79

Go into the main area of a hospital   84

Go into an empty hospital waiting room   92

~~Sit in the waiting area at my doctor's office   94~~   (doing empty hospital instead)

~~Go to the drug store pharmacy area   63~~   (doing parking lot instead)

~~Sit in an emergency room waiting area   100~~   (doing busy hospital instead)

~~Visit a trauma unit~~ (no trauma unit in my city)

Go into a busy hospital waiting room where   100
    there are many sick people

FIGURE 8. **Things related to Francis's fear of catching a disease from being near sick people.**

from sick people. This was a becoming a big problem, because he couldn't bring himself to visit his friends and family when they were in the hospital. He set up a series of exercises, starting with the one he was least anxious about and ending with the one he was most anxious about. His exercises looked like this:

1. Walk past a hospital (initial anxiety rating = 53)
2. Walk through a hospital parking lot (initial anxiety rating = 64)
3. Walk up to a hospital entrance (initial anxiety rating = 79)

4. *Go into the main area of a hospital (initial anxiety rating = 84)*
5. *Go into an empty hospital waiting room (initial anxiety rating = 92)*
6. *Go into a busy hospital waiting room where there are many sick people (initial anxiety rating = 100)*

Step 3: Practice Your Exposure Exercises. As with the interoceptive exposure exercises, the situational exercises should be brief and should be practiced daily. We recommend that you move from one exercise to the next on your list only after your anxiety ratings have dropped by at least 20 on the 1-to-100 rating scale. Don't rush! Stay with the activity long enough *during one practice of the exercise* for the anxiety it causes to decrease. Francis took 20 minutes a day over a three-week period to work through his series of exercises. He monitored his progress every day. After walking past a neighborhood hospital for 10 minutes, his anxiety rating dropped from 53 to 20. The next day he walked through the hospital parking lot two times for 10 minutes each time. Again his anxiety dropped by more than 20 points. The last four exercises were more difficult, taking between two and five days each to work through. Despite a strong desire to avoid the last four situations, Francis forced himself to experience the anxiety they provoked until it started to decline. Although he was still somewhat anxious at the end of the three weeks of practice, Francis was actually able to go visit a close friend in the hospital. His anxiety rating during the hospital visit was 50.

In some cases you may notice that tackling and overcoming the situations that cause you the most health anxiety will reduce your anxiety for other activities or situations as well. If your second- and third-ranked situations continue to make you anxious, repeat Steps 2 and 3 for each one until your anxiety decreases.

Monitor Your Exposure Progress

Use Worksheet 13 to keep track of each exposure exercise you do, when you do it, how anxious it makes you feel, and what you learn from doing it. As with previous exercises, you might find it helpful to make a chart of your anxiety ratings. We recommend that you make a chart to compare your pre-exercise anxiety ratings for your top three feared bodily sensations or situations with the ratings you make on Worksheet 13 after practicing each exercise. If the exposure exercises you selected were effective, you should see an overall decrease in the amount of anxiety each bodily sensation or situation made you feel. This may take anywhere from several days to a few weeks. You should also be able to add to your evidence for the alternative explanations you listed on Worksheet 8 from Chapter 6. For example, for the alternative explanation "the lumps in my breasts are harmless cysts," a person might add "repeated poking and prodding of breast tissue increases pain and swelling, whereas leaving it alone reduces it."

At times you may be tempted to turn to any security blankets you have for comfort from feelings of fear and anxiety brought on during practice of your interoceptive and situational exposure exercises. Try your hardest not to give in to this temptation. Remind yourself that you want to let the stress reaction happen, that feelings of anxiety associated with the stress reaction aren't harmful, and that they'll pass within a few minutes or so. If you do give in, make a note of this on Worksheet 13 and try working through the exercises described next as a way of letting go of your security blankets.

Letting Go of Security Blankets

Many of our patients use security blankets as a way of coping with their health anxiety. We can't overstate how important it is that you try to let your security blankets go. Easier said than done? Maybe not. Many people find it next to impossible to go "cold turkey" but have success when they have a little help.

This help comes in the form of small modifications to the exercises you've already learned for testing the effectiveness of checking and reassurance-seeking behaviors. Matt, for example, worked through three steps very similar to those described for overcoming checking and reassurance seeking so he could stop carrying around his nitroglycerin pills. First, he listed the advantages and disadvantages of carrying the pills. He noted feeling safe as an advantage but now understood how this behavior fed his health anxiety. Second, he came up with a few alternatives—he could stop carrying the pills altogether, he could keep them nearby but not in his pockets, or he could increase their presence by putting them in his line of sight at all times. He decided to try going without carrying the pills for three days. His anxiety didn't drop much. In fact, he felt more anxious, feeling he'd most certainly die without the pills if the "big one" happened. Next he tried putting a bottle of pills where he could see them almost all of the time—on his night table, beside his toothbrush, in his car, on his computer monitor at work, and on top of the refrigerator at home. Over a three-day period he came to realize that the pills really did cause him to worry more about his health and, to his surprise, that this worry was what made him feel he needed the pills handy "just in case." Finally, when he tried again to go without carrying the pills, his anxiety about not having them handy dropped from a rating of 90 to one of 50 in two days. Try modifying the three steps for overcoming checking and reassurance seeking in order to identify and work toward letting go of your security blankets.

There is no special key to deciding in what order to test your alternatives to using your security blankets; it's just a matter of trying different alternatives. Eventually (and fairly quickly) you'll be able to show yourself that your security blankets keep your anxiety alive and that you're safe without them.

Coping with Fear of Death

Worries about bodily sensations or catching horrific diseases are usually related to a fear of death. Some people with health anxiety can think of almost nothing but death and what it holds for them. They're constantly worried about dying, and they often wonder whether their uncomfortable bodily sensations will go on for eternity after they die: "Death won't bring me any relief. I'm probably going to lie in my grave with this excruciating and incessant head pain forever."

Worrying a lot about death is similar to some of the other health-related worries we've talked about in that it feeds the health anxiety cycle. But it's different in a very important way. How is it different from worrying that muscle weakness is due to multiple sclerosis or that chest pain signals an oncoming heart attack? How is it different from worrying that you'll catch an infectious disease by using public washrooms? It's different from these worries because there isn't an alternative explanation to the thought that "I'm going to die." It's a fact of life that we're all going to die someday. It's inevitable.

Many of the strategies we've introduced to you in this chapter are designed to help you make life richer and more enjoyable; but they won't work to their fullest potential if you spend most of your time worrying about death and dying. The good news (although it may not sound all that good) is that the fear of death can also be overcome by facing it head on. We've all heard stories or seen movies about people who've brushed shoulders with death and come away with a renewed appreciation for all that life has to offer. We can't directly expose you to death and have you come back having learned from your experience. But you can try the following:

- Prepare a will.
- Read the obituary section of your local newspaper.
- Visit cemeteries and read the inscriptions on the headstones.
- Visit funeral homes to enquire about the type, availability, and cost of funeral services.
- Write a detailed description of your death. Do this by hand rather than on a computer or typewriter and don't worry about spelling or grammar. Include as much information as possible about your death—how it feels, what it sounds like, what you're thinking at the time, what emotions you have—and the aftermath that you're afraid of. Read the description back to yourself.
- Write your own obituary.

These exercises are based on the same principles as the interoceptive and situational exposure exercises you've already learned; that is, they're meant to be repeated until the anxiety they provoke becomes less and less. The goal isn't to make you happy about death but, rather, to help you face it without too much worry. You can use Worksheet 13 to track the exercises you perform, your anxiety at the time, and what you learn.

Things to Remember

There's an important lesson to be learned from each of these exercises: Behaviors that we know keep health anxiety alive can be overcome. You can beat them. Sometimes it does take a while to learn the lesson that will help you break your health anxiety cycle. For this reason we recommend that you keep track of the details of all the exercises you do—when you do them, what you do, how much anxiety you feel, and what you learn. This will allow you to see how you're progressing. Make copies of Worksheet 13 and use it to keep track of these things. You can make graphs like those from Chapters 5 and 6, if you like, to chart your progress. With consistent practice you'll see results in three weeks. But it's important to keep practicing the things you learn on a daily basis. This will help keep your health anxiety at bay.

These exercises will challenge you. Constantly remind yourself of the good reasons that you're working on these exercises—breaking your health anxiety cycle and taking back control of your life. Reward yourself for small successes: Congratulate yourself and treat yourself to something you enjoy. Sometimes things will be smooth sailing, and you'll steadily become less and less frightened. At other times things may get a little rough, and progress may be more like one step forward and two steps back. You might become a little more comfortable about your feared bodily sensations or situations, only to experience an increase again. Francis was feeling much less anxious around sick people, but then one day, while visiting a cousin in the hospital, he felt a return of his anxiety to levels he hadn't experienced in a while. He stayed to visit his cousin despite the increasing anxiety, but he did excuse himself early. The next day he started working through his exposure exercises again, and, within a week, he was visiting his cousin without much anxiety. Flare-ups like this will occur from time to time. Simple strategies for dealing with flare-ups are outlined in Chapter 10.

If things get tough, remember that persistence pays off. You can also remind yourself that:

• You're investing some short-term pain for the payoff of long-term gain—taking back control of your life and learning to live it without too much health anxiety.
• You need to come face to face with your fears to overcome them. If you get anxious while doing exercises designed to change the behaviors that feed your health anxiety, it means you're doing the right things. Use the relaxation

and breathing retraining exercises when your anxiety increases to the point of getting out of control.

• Some days will be better than others. You're going to have days when everything seems to be working and when your health anxiety seems under control. Great! You'll also have bad days. Don't let these get you down. Lance Armstrong, a testicular cancer survivor and now an astounding six-time winner of the Tour de France, put it this way:

> If I had a bad day, I had a tendency to say "Well, I've just been through three surgeries, three months of chemo, and a year of hell, and that's the reason I'm not riding well. My body is just never going to be the same." But what I really should have been saying was "Hey, it's just a bad day." (L. Armstrong with S. Jenkins, 2002, *It's not about the bike: My journey back to life.* New York: G. P. Putnam's Sons, p. 188)

Part III

MAINTAINING YOUR GAINS

Eight

Dealing with Doctors

We all visit the doctor from time to time. But people with health anxiety tend to visit their doctors more frequently. Some have excellent relationships with their doctors, but others don't. How is your relationship with the doctors you visit about your health concerns? Answering the following questions will give you a good idea.

- Do you often have problems dealing with doctors?
- Are they rude or angry with you?
- Does it seem that they dismiss your concerns or don't care?
- Do you sometimes think your doctors don't take your problems seriously?
- Do you sometimes feel your doctors don't really want to talk to you about your problems?
- Do you find they can't help you?

If you answered *yes* to any of these questions, your relationship with your doctors apparently isn't at its best. This chapter is for you. Our goal is to help you gain a better understanding of the kinds of relationships that people with health anxiety have with their doctors. We'll also suggest a few strategies that you can use to improve things between you and your doctors.

Here are some examples to illustrate the sorts of doctor–patient problems that we're talking about.

Joanne: "Why is the doctor ignoring me?"

Joanne goes to the hospital ER because she has a pain in her right side. She's worried that there's something wrong with one of her kidneys.

The doctor peeks into the waiting area and sees Joanne. He rolls his eyes, and she thinks she hears him mutter under his breath, "Not you again." This is Joanne's fifth trip to the ER in the past month, each for different health concerns. On this visit, the doctor leaves Joanne in the waiting room for several hours. Other patients come and go while she sits waiting. The doctor doesn't come, even though Joanne complains a number of times to the receptionist. Frustrated and angry, Joanne storms out, vowing never to go to that ER again.

Weihong: "Are they all incompetent?"

Weihong wants to be absolutely certain that there's nothing wrong with his heart. He notices that it sometimes skips a beat and fears that there's something seriously wrong. Weihong's family doctor couldn't find anything wrong with his heart. And yet the doctor couldn't say with 100-percent certainty that there was nothing wrong. This frightened Weihong, so he went from doctor to doctor to be absolutely certain that his heart was healthy. Although the doctors generally agreed that Weihong's heart was fine, they gave vague and sometimes conflicting information about the causes of skipped beats. As a result, Weihong felt confused and even more frightened. He believed that maybe his doctors weren't sufficiently competent to diagnose his sort of heart problem.

Warren: "He says it's all in my head."

Warren enters a small consulting room to see his family doctor. The doctor looks tired and distracted. Warren has a long list of health concerns. He knows that time is short so he describes his problems as quickly and in as much detail as he can. It seems to Warren that he's only just started listing his problems when his doctor sighs and scribbles something on a prescription pad. Interrupting Warren in mid-sentence, the doctor tells him that he's just suffering from "nerves." As the doctor leaves to see his next patient he hands Warren a prescription for a tranquilizer.

Jasminder: "I'll find another doctor, then."

Jasminder sits anxiously by her telephone, awaiting the results of her latest medical test. For some weeks she'd been feeling tired and had a sick feeling in her stomach. Her doctor couldn't find anything wrong with Jasminder. The doctor said it was probably just stress, but she'd perform some lab tests just to be sure. A week later, the doctor called. Jasminder jumped nervously at the shrill ring of the phone. The tests were negative, and Jasminder was told that she had nothing to worry about. But Jasminder continued to worry; she felt tired and sickly and her doctor couldn't tell her why. She picked up the phone book and began searching for another doctor who could give her more tests.

Diagnosing Your Doctor Problems

It's more likely than not that you've had an interaction with your doctor like one of those just described. To help you nail down the source of your problems with doctors, please read the following list and check off all that apply to you.

☐ Doctors don't listen to me.

☐ They get mad at me.

☐ They make fun of my problems.

☐ They don't tell me what's causing my problems.

☐ They're not available when I need to talk to them.

☐ They don't believe me when I describe my symptoms.

☐ They tell me my problems are "all in my head."

☐ They aren't able to tell me, with 100-percent certainty, that I'm healthy.

☐ They don't examine me properly.

☐ They don't perform enough medical tests.

Notice that we've already talked about some of these things in earlier chapters. For example, you know that what you're feeling in your body isn't all in your head. The sensations and changes might not be from disease, but many of them are caused by something very real—your body's response to stress. Knowing this will give you the confidence you need to challenge any doctor who suggests that the things you're visiting about are simply all in your head. You'll be able to help them better understand how the body's stress reaction can cause bodily sensations and changes that mimic some diseases. You've also learned that the need for absolute certainty is an unrealistic way of thinking that can be changed and that medical tests aren't needed to explain many of the things you've been worried about. Later in this chapter we'll talk about some other things you can do to deal with these problems. But, first, let's consider why things can go wrong in the relationship between you and your doctor.

Who's to Blame?

Whose "fault" is it when things go wrong in the doctor–patient relationship? This is a question we commonly hear. But, in our view, this isn't the right question to be asking. Blame doesn't solve the problem; it only makes people feel guilty, angry, or resentful. A more helpful question is "How can I better understand and overcome the problems I have with my doctors?" Sure, sometimes the problem might lie with your doctors. Just like other professions, the medical profession has its share of the good, the good enough, and the not so good. If you've been unlucky enough to have an incompetent doctor, then by all means seek another medical professional. But, if you've had problems with many different doctors, then maybe the problem lies in the way you and your doctors interact. In other words, the problem may not be the doctor but, instead, the *relationship* between you and the doctor.

To make the best use of your doctors, it's important for you to know two things. First, you need to understand the sorts of doctor–patient relationships that doctors do and don't enjoy. Second, it will help to know the things you can do to make sure that you get the most out of your interactions with doctors.

Put Yourself in the Doctor's Shoes

No two doctors are alike, but there are some things that many doctors prefer. They like to be able to solve problems, to fix things. Imagine how satisfying it feels to be able to diagnose and cure a serious disease. Now imagine how frustrating it must feel to have patients that you can't help—patients who return again and again, complaining of symptoms you can't cure. This is how many doctors feel about patients with health anxiety disorders.

Family doctors, who are usually overworked and under pressure to get through a long list of patients, often don't have the time or expertise to treat health anxiety. In a bid to do something helpful, they might simply try to reassure their patients who have excessive health anxiety that there's nothing physically wrong with them. Or they might order more medical tests to appease the anxious patient (or their own fear of missing a physical problem). But, as we discussed in previous chapters, giving reassurance and ordering unnecessary medical tests can make health anxiety worse. People with health anxiety become addicted to reassurance. And unnecessary medical tests can put people at risk of harmful effects (for example, scarring and pain from repeated exploratory surgeries) or complications that sometimes happen with invasive medical procedures. When it comes to treating health anxiety, doctors often need to do the opposite of what they usually do, as captured in the saying "Don't just do something, stand there!" That is, sometimes the things they do are more harmful than helpful.

So, how does this information help you? It tells you that doctors are pretty good at identifying and treating physical problems. But, for people with anxiety-based concerns, such as health anxiety, many doctors, particularly family doctors, don't have the time or expertise to give helpful assistance or treatment. Sometimes they refer their health anxious patients to a specialist, such as a psychologist or psychiatrist. This doesn't mean that they believe the symptoms reported by their patients aren't real. In fact, the doctors who refer their health-anxious patients to mental health professionals are usually the ones who really *do* understand that their symptoms are real. They're the ones who know that your concerns require specialized treatment along the lines of what we've discussed in Part 2 of this book.

The problem is that many people with health anxiety stubbornly refuse to see a psychologist or psychiatrist. They worry that people will think they're crazy because they're seeing a "shrink." It's quite likely that you felt this way, even if only a little, when you started reading Chapter 1. It may be helpful to know that, over the past decade, the stigma associated with anxiety-related health problems has greatly lessened. Movie stars and other celebrities often appear on TV or in magazines talking about their struggles with different anxiety disorders. It's a sign of wisdom to be able to see the right specialist. If you're suffering from severe anxiety about your health, then you owe it to yourself to seek help, regardless of whether you have a serious disease or whether you're perfectly healthy. (People with life-threatening health problems, such as cancer, are often anxious, and part of their treatment involves specific therapies for anxiety.) If you continue to be bothered by a lot of health anxiety after working through the exercises in this book, we strongly recommend that you see a psychologist or psychiatrist who specializes in health-anxiety disorders to discuss your concerns. We'll talk about this further in Chapter 10.

Getting the Most Out of Your Doctors

Even people with health anxiety get sick occasionally. You might have heard the joke about the hypochondriac's gravestone, which read, "See—I told you I was ill!" So, even if you decide to see a specialist for health anxiety, you'll still need to figure out how to get the most out of your interactions with your family doctor. Here are some useful *dos* and *don'ts* to keep in mind.

Dos include the following:

• Ask yourself "Do I really need to see a doctor right now?" What is your doctor likely to tell you? Many people with health anxiety already know what their doctor will say; for example, "There's nothing wrong with you; you're simply experiencing anxiety symptoms." Try delaying your medical appointment for a week to see if you can get control of your troubling symptoms by working through the strategies you've learned in this book. If the symptoms don't go away after a week, make an appointment with your doctor.

• If you decide to see a doctor, try to be clear about why you're there and what you want her or him to do for you.

• In the past, some doctors may not have given you the respect you deserve. Unfortunately, it happens. But try to take responsibility for your contribution to problems in the doctor–patient relationship. If you're angry or rude to your doctor, he or she might become angry or avoid you as a result. Nobody likes to be around angry, demanding people. Instead, use the things you've learned from earlier chapters in this book to have relaxed and informed discussions about your concerns.

• Consider seeing a mental health specialist. They can help you understand and overcome any lingering health anxiety you have. (Most doctors' offices have pamphlets or referral information on the agencies or individuals who can help with mental health problems. We've also provided a partial list of specialists at the back of this book.)

• Give yourself credit for thinking about how you can improve your relationship with your doctor. It's a problem to be solved. Try to set aside any anger or guilt as you analyze the problem. The problem-solving strategies covered in Chapter 5 may be useful here.

• Let your doctor know you have a tendency to worry about your health and thank him or her for the time and attention given to you. Your doctor will appreciate this.

Don'ts include:

• Don't overwhelm your doctor with too much information. Frustrated doctors sometimes refer to the information overload as the "organ recital." Pick your *main problem* and describe that to your doctor (see *Dos*). If you like, write your other problems down on a sheet of paper to give to your doctor.

• Don't demand 100-percent certainty. No medical test is completely accurate. Remember that we all have to accept that life is full of uncertainties. A stray satellite could fall through your roof while you're reading this book. An earthquake could suddenly swallow you up. An out-of-control truck could suddenly crash into your house. These are all unlikely, but there is no 100-guarantee that they won't happen. Like it or not, we all have to accept that life is filled with uncertainties.

• Don't repeatedly seek reassurance. As you know, reassurance is addictive; you can never get enough. By repeatedly seeking medical reassurance, you put yourself in a position in which you feel dependent and constantly worried. And your doctor will probably get frustrated if you repeatedly ask for reassurance.

• Don't go "doctor shopping." Find a doctor who is good enough and stick with him or her. The overwhelming majority of doctors are good enough.

- The emergency room is for emergencies. Don't go there unless you really have to. If you're having sudden and clearly unusual signs or symptoms (for example, bleeding from the rectum, persistent vomiting) then a visit to the emergency room may be in order. If the signs and symptoms are similar to things you've experienced before, see if you can gain control of them with the relaxation and breathing exercises you've learned. This will help in many cases. If not, ask yourself if you could wait to see your family doctor instead of going to the emergency room.

Things to Remember

It's very common for people with health anxiety to have problems in their dealings with doctors. You might feel demeaned and not believed (or dismissed), and your doctor may feel angry or frustrated. It's important to remember that there are many things you can do—and can refrain from doing—that will help you make the best use of your doctors. Analyze the problem and try some of the strategies suggested in this chapter. If, after working through the strategies you've learned for breaking the health anxiety cycle, you continue feeling tempted to see your doctor almost every time you notice noise in your body, one of the best solutions may involve making an appointment to see a psychologist or psychiatrist who specializes in the health anxiety disorders. And, finally, keep in mind that there are times when it is important to see your doctor.

When Should I Seek Medical Attention?

"When should I go to my doctor?" This is a good question that we hear all the time from our patients. Here we are, advising you to cut down on your doctor visits, and you're probably wondering when you really ought to seek medical attention. There certainly are times when you should do so. You and your doctor together could generate a list of reasons for seeking medical attention. This list will depend on your physical health and medical history. If you are elderly or have a serious illness, you might need to have regularly *scheduled* medical appointments, for example, every two weeks. Because everyone is different and has differing medical needs, we recommend that you discuss this with your doctor. Worksheet 15 can be used to get this discussion going with your doctor.

Here are some examples of times when you should go ahead and see your family doctor:

- When new, painful symptoms develop (for example, chest pain).
- When you experience bodily sensations or changes that are clearly not normal and don't appear to be part of the stress reaction (for example, blood in the urine, loss of continence, inability to speak).

Worksheet 15. When to Visit the Doctor

Instructions: Answer the questions below. Make an appointment with your doctor to discuss the things you've listed. Have him or her assist you in completing the list of confirmed medical illnesses that you should keep an eye on. Working together, come up with a list of times when you should visit the doctor.

Write down all anxiety-related bodily sensations or changes you have. Looking back at worksheets from other chapters may help.

Write down any bodily sensations or symptoms you have that you haven't been able to explain.

What confirmed medical illness do you have? Are regular check-ups for any of these necessary? List check-up frequency for each.

(cont.)

List all legitimate reasons for seeing your doctor here.

I'll visit my family doctor at these times:

- When I have a scheduled annual medical examination.

- When I need inoculations.

- If I need to renew a prescription.

- When I experience bodily sensations that are clearly not normal and don't seem to be part of the stress reaction (for example, blood in my urine, loss of continence, inability to speak).

- _____

- _____

- _____

- _____

- _____

- _____

- _____

- _____

- _____

- _____

- _____

- When the symptoms of your chronic, medically confirmed diseases flare up and thereby warrant medical intervention (for example, worsening of diabetes or colitis).
- When you need an annual medical examination or inoculation (for example, mammography, prostate exam, flu shot).
- When you need to renew a prescription medication. (In some states or provinces, patients can't phone in their renewals and need to make an appointment to see their doctor in order to get this done.)

These are examples of good reasons for visiting your doctor. Evaluate your *specific* reasons whenever you feel the need to see your doctor. If these reasons are not on the preceding list, try writing the reason down, putting off the visit, and reassessing the need for going to the doctor in a week. Practice the strategies you've learned for dealing with your health anxiety. In many cases, you'll notice that the things that prompted you to want to go to the doctor a week earlier are no longer of current concern. That is, you'll have demonstrated your control over your health anxiety by reaffirming that bodily sensations and changes that cause you to worry can actually come and go without being harmful.

Gavin: "Now I'm moving and grooving."

Gavin was in his seventies. Although he was fairly healthy for his age, he worried a lot about his health. He sought reassurance from his doctor each week and often phoned in-between appointments for more reassurance. His doctor became resentful and annoyed at the repeated interruptions, to the point that the doctor was not returning Gavin's calls. This made Gavin even more anxious, because it looked like his doctor was not taking proper care of him. During the weekly medical appointments, Gavin gave a long, rambling account of his many health concerns. His doctor felt helpless and overwhelmed and came to dread their weekly appointments.

Reluctantly, Gavin agreed to see a psychologist for his health anxiety. Much to his surprise, he found the psychological therapy to be helpful. The therapist had plenty of time to listen to him, and she appeared to be genuinely concerned about his suffering. Gavin was encouraged to make better use of his medical consultations. He wrote out his health concerns beforehand and gave the list to the doctor. Gavin also worked at being more to the point in what he said to his doctor, focusing on his most important health concern. He was also encouraged to delay or refrain from seeking reassurance. This enabled him to learn that his worrisome symptoms simply came and went, without any harmful consequences. As Gavin came to be less demanding with his doctor, the doctor–patient relationship improved. On those rare occasions that he did phone for advice, Gavin's calls were promptly returned. The doctor no longer dreaded their appointments.

Gavin's health anxiety gradually lessened, and he became physically more active. For example, he took daily walks in a nearby park. In his own words, he was "moving and grooving" instead of staying home worrying about his health. As the psychological therapy came to an end, Gavin raised the important questions of when and how often he should consult his family doctor. Gavin, his doctor, and his psychologist drew up a set of guidelines that included the aforementioned reasons for seeking medical attention. Gavin and his family doctor also agreed that he would have check-ups every four weeks and that he would phone the doctor only when absolutely necessary, and not simply for reassurance. Gavin was satisfied with the plan and felt that his health was being properly cared for.

Nine

Helping Friends and Family Help You

Friends and family members of people with health anxiety commonly ask us such questions as, "What can I do to help him overcome his health anxiety?" and "What can I do to cope with living with someone who's always worrying about being sick? I know it doesn't help, but I can't stop myself from getting frustrated." Undoubtedly, you've had a variety of reactions from people who know that you worry a lot about your health. Some may have been reassuring, some might have tried giving you advice, some may have become annoyed or angry about your concerns, and some may have simply brushed you off as being concerned over nothing. It's not unusual for the same person to react in different ways at different times. The truth is that your health anxiety has affected both you and those who care about you; and, in turn, the way they treat you has influenced your health anxiety. This chapter will help you understand two things: how your health anxiety has affected the important people in your life and why they react to you the way they do. With this understanding you'll be in a better position to help your family and friends learn what they can do to assist you in breaking your health anxiety cycle.

Most people who spend a lot of time with a person who has health anxiety experience one of two reactions: They tend to become either *stressed out* or *overinvolved*. Think about the important people in your life. Do some of them seem to be tense and on edge around you? Are others always trying to help? Let's take a look at each of these reactions in more detail. While reading through the next few sections, keep in mind that our intention is not to blame you or those who care about you. Our goal is to help you understand these reactions and how they affect your relationships so that you can teach family and friends how they can help you.

The Stressed-Out Loved One

Katy: "It's not fair that I have to listen."

Katy was at the end of her rope. Her relationship with her sister Andrea had become increasingly strained over the past several months. It seemed that every time they got together Andrea would complain incessantly about her health and would ask Katy for advice, help, or reassurance. Katy had gone along with it for a while. In fact, she'd even taken time off work to drive Andrea to several doctors' appointments. But her patience was wearing thin. This week while they were having coffee, Andrea worried that her eyelids were twitching. "Are my eyelids twitching?" she would repeatedly ask. "Not that I can see," sighed Katy. "Do you think it's just stress?" asked Andrea. "Probably." What Katy thought and really wanted to say was "I wish you'd stop this preoccupation with your health—it's not fair that I have to listen to this every time we get together." Katy held her tongue, but the irritation grew. Andrea went on and on about her health concerns. Finally, Katy couldn't take it anymore. "I need to go," she snapped. Getting up, Katy stormed out of the coffee shop, leaving Andrea feeling hurt, alone, and bewildered.

Your health anxiety can extend beyond you and be stressful to others. Although most people are genuinely concerned for you, they do very often have to put up with repeated pleas for reassurance: "Do I look pale?" "Feel my forehead. Do you think I have a temperature?" "Do you think this freckle looks unusual?" Some find themselves drawn into a caretaking role, chauffeuring you to and from medical appointments and taking over extra household responsibilities ("I'm too weak to take out the trash. You'll have to do it for me").

The extra demands placed on them frequently lead those close to you to feel frustrated and resentful. They may react by criticizing you: "Will you *please* stop whining about your aches and pains. I can't stand it anymore!" Or they may resort to nagging to make you stop worrying about your health: "Jason, stop griping about your stomachaches. You know it's only stress. Get out of bed and get ready for school, this instant!"

When stressed-out loved ones of a person with health anxiety come to see us, we ask them about the things they try to do to help. We hear all sorts of answers, but there are some common themes. Often they will grudgingly go along with requests made of them ("Okay, Andrea, I'll take you to the ER again, even though you bloody well know the doctor will tell you—again—that there's nothing wrong with you"). As they go along with more and more requests, resentment and anger build, to the point that they may have an angry outburst

("Goddamn it, Bob, for the hundredth time I can't see anything wrong with your tongue!"). The angry outburst may be followed by feelings of guilt ("I'm sorry, honey, that I blew up at you because you were worried about the color of your tongue"). This is usually followed by more requests for reassurance by the person with health anxiety and by resentment building yet again. Thus the stressed-out relative or friend may be caught in his or her own vicious cycle—a cycle of building resentment, anger outbursts, guilt, and then more resentment. In an effort to break the cycle, he or she may avoid the person with health anxiety, leaving that person feeling hurt and abandoned.

Some stressed-out loved ones take a different approach; they resort to constant nagging in an effort to get the person with health anxiety to stop acting like an invalid: "Mary, for the third time, will you get out of bed and feed the kids their breakfast. I've got to go to work!" Nagging often doesn't work. In fact, it can make things worse. Nagging causes tension and stress over being nagged and thereby increases stress-related bodily reactions (for example, headaches, stomach upset, hot flashes), which feed health anxiety. So what's the next resort? Often it's even *more* nagging, on the notion that if a little bit doesn't work, maybe a lot is needed." Unfortunately, this escalates the problem, straining relationships and increasing everyone's stress reaction. Nobody benefits.

The Overinvolved Loved One

> *Bill: "It's my duty as a good spouse."*
>
> Bill prided himself on being a loyal, devoted husband. Whenever Emily complained of feeling ill, he fussed about, trying to make her as comfortable as possible. Sometimes he went off to the drugstore in search of remedies; on other occasions he rushed her to the doctor. Lately, Emily was suffering from headaches. She worried she might have a brain tumor. Bill took her to see many doctors about the headaches. Each time the doctors said they were due to stress. Emily wasn't convinced, so Bill volunteered to search the Internet for possible causes of headaches. The information he retrieved was truly alarming. Emily and Bill learned of all kinds of rare, lethal causes of headaches. This alarmed Emily even more and, in fact, seemed to trigger more headaches. After that, whenever Emily complained of a headache, she asked Bill whether he thought she should go to the ER. He knew that the headaches were probably due to stress, but he thought it was his duty as a good husband to make sure that Emily got the best possible medical attention, so he usually took her to the ER.

Some well-meaning friends and family members may be willing to do just about anything for you—take you to medical appointments, pick up your prescriptions, offer reassurance, and assume all household responsibilities. Sometimes, as in Bill's case, overinvolved family and friends will even scour the newspapers and Internet for information relevant to your health concerns: "John, I know you're worried about toxins in the food, so I checked the Internet for information on which foods to avoid." "Maria, you said you're frightened of airborne viruses, so I've picked up some information on the best sorts of face masks to use."

Why do some people become overinvolved with health anxiety? In our experience there are two main reasons. First, the person may take on this role because of a well-meaning sense of duty: "I love my husband, so I need to look after him." Although they may have the best of intentions, overinvolved family and friends may be doing you more harm than good. Indeed, needless doting on you can make your problems worse. It can:

- Reinforce the false message that you are frail and sickly, and
- Encourage you to needlessly become an invalid, lying on the couch all day, focusing on your body, and worrying about your health, when, instead, you should be up and about, actively engaged in living life to the fullest.

Second, your loved one may actually enjoy looking after you. Taking care of another person is an important task that makes us all feel needed and important. Your loved one may not necessarily be aware of this as a reason that he or she attends to your every need. It could be part of a lifelong habit of looking after people. As we've said before, your loved one is not to blame, nor are you. People are drawn into patterns of behavior for all sorts of reasons. The important thing is for people to become aware of the consequences of their behavior and to try new behaviors if need be.

What Roles Do Your Loved Ones Play?

Think about the people you usually spend time with—your spouse or partner, your kids, a parent, a brother or sister, your best friend, other important people in your life. Answer these questions for each person close to you. Do they:

☐ Often feel resentful or annoyed toward you?

☐ Become outwardly angry with you?

☐ Try to avoid you?

☐ Feel guilty or apologetic after getting angry with you?

☐ Nag you so you'll stop complaining?

☐ Offer you all the reassurance they can?

☐ Collect information about the disease that you're worried about?

☐ Take over most or all of your chores and other responsibilities?

☐ Drive you to doctors' appointments?

☐ Offer to get medicines or other remedies for you at the pharmacy?

If most of your check marks fall on some or all of the first five options, then your loved one is likely stressed out. If most of your check marks were placed on some or all of the last five options, then your loved one may be overinvolved. If you checked several of the first and last five options, then your loved one may be both stressed out *and* overinvolved. Knowing what roles your loved ones have adopted when interacting with you and your health anxiety will allow you to help them change in a way that will help you break your health anxiety cycle.

How to Help Them Help You

There are several basic things you can do to help your family and friends help you conquer your health anxiety. You can start by suggesting that they read the other chapters in this book so they, too, have a better understanding of health anxiety, its causes, and the strategies that you've been learning for overcoming it. They can benefit from reading this chapter. We find that when the family and friend of a person with health anxiety have a better understanding of what health anxiety is, they're in a better position to identify the helpful things they can do. And they're better able to avoid doing things that make health anxiety worse (the things you checked off as things your loved ones do when interacting with you).

You can also spend some time together talking about reassurance seeking and its role in health anxiety. It's really important that those close to you understand how reassurance plays into your health anxiety cycle. You can use the strategies in Chapter 8 to stop seeking reassurance from loved ones, but your success in breaking the health anxiety cycle will be limited if they don't stop giving it to you. Think of it as similar to trying to quit smoking. If cigarettes aren't kept handy, many people who quit smoking can successfully go without. But many times all it takes for them to give in to temptation and start smoking again is for someone to offer a cigarette. You need to let your family and friends know that people with health anxiety are more or less *addicted* to seeking reassurance. They also need to understand that although the immediate effect of giving you reassurance is one of calming, it's also one of the things that keep your health anxiety alive in the long run. Sit down with your family and friends and explain these things to them. Ask them if they understand, and work on it until they do. We recommend that you work out an agreement wherein you promise not to seek reassurance and they promise not to give it, whether asked for or not. Figure 9 may be helpful in discussing the effects of reassurance and in agreeing to "kick it."

Katy: "Can we talk about something else?"

Katy and Andrea resumed meeting for coffee some time after Andrea had been in therapy for her health anxiety. Compared with the way she had been previously, Andrea seemed more relaxed, and her discussion with Katy was more like a true conversation. For Katy, this was a wel-

---

Giving me reassurance, although done out of caring and a desire to help, can actually make my health anxiety worse. There are a few ways reassurance can do this.

- It can increase my preoccupation with disease by extending the amount of time I dwell on my bodily sensations and changes. It feeds my health anxiety by giving some temporary relief that is followed by even more anxiety.

- When I'm repeatedly given reassurance, there's a chance that I'll eventually be exposed to alarming information about rare but lethal diseases. For example, if you tell me that everything is okay and that my symptoms are probably just the result of some minor ailment or change in my day-to-day routine, I'll probably feel better for a while. But when the symptoms come back, I'll probably dismiss your reassurance and go look for some other cause. So by giving me reassurance you can make me even more anxious about my health.

- Giving me repeated reassurance can make me feel vulnerable, helpless, and dependent. By having turned to you for help in the past, I may have actually "trained" you to inquire about my health and to offer me assurances. Doing this makes me feel better for a while, but in the long run it makes me feel more helpless and reinforces the belief that I'm weak and vulnerable.

If we could agree on two things, it would really help me succeed in taking back my life from health anxiety. Can we agree that (1) I'll try not to seek reassurance from you about my health, and (2) you'll try not to give it when I ask or at any other time. Instead, you can say something like, "Sorry, honey, but its doctor's orders that I don't reassure you."

FIGURE 9. **The harmful effects of giving reassurance.**

come relief from their previous get-togethers, which consisted of monologues from Andrea about her health. Although Andrea's health anxiety was much better, she occasionally lapsed into reassurance seeking. It was a habit that was hard to break. At one point over coffee, Andrea mentioned that she'd been feeling chilly that morning. "Do you think I look pale?" asked Andrea. Katy replied, "Andrea, as you know, we're not supposed to discuss your health. It only makes your anxiety worse. Can we talk about something else?" Andrea replied, "Okay, sorry, I know. Sometimes it's hard to break the habit." "Let's talk about that new job of yours," replied Katy.

Even well-meaning inquiries from loved ones, such as "How are you feeling?" or "How ya doing today?" can cause your attention to drift to issues of health. Make an agreement not to discuss your health. This may be easy in some cases and more difficult in others. Stressed-out family members and friends usually welcome this kind of arrangement with open arms. On the other hand, it's often difficult for overinvolved loved ones to find a way to shift from what's been an almost all-consuming focus on your health worries to something completely different. It helps to develop a relationship around positive things unrelated to illness. For example, rather than talking about your health, you might talk about movies, current events, and the most enjoyable activities of the day. People find pleasure in reconnecting through common interests.

Cognitive-behavioral therapists encourage people with health anxiety to pursue active, fulfilling lifestyles (for example, taking the dog for a daily walk instead of lying in bed dwelling on your health). Involve your loved ones in some of the things you enjoy doing. This will give you a chance to spend quality time together, may give you another shared interest to chat about, and will provide you with a source of encouragement at times when you're not feeling overly motivated and need that little nudge to get off your butt.

Specific Advice for Stressed-Out Family and Friends

There are more specific things that your stressed-out family and friends can do to help you succeed in overcoming your health anxiety. We've found it most helpful to summarize these things in a list of *dos* and *don'ts* with examples that can be shared with those close to you. Think of these *dos* and *don'ts* as guidelines rather than rigid rules. Again, we suggest that you sit down with your loved ones and discuss these things with them. They need to try these things out and use their best judgment as to which things work for them.

1. "*Do* try to understand why I'm worried about my health and how my anxiety feeds itself. With better understanding you'll be less likely to blame me for the difficulties I've had overcoming my worries. You'll be better able to help me put things into perspective."

   Example: Jim's wife was able to reframe her annoyance into a response that assisted Jim in gathering evidence against his specific thought that he'd die of heart failure.

   "Jim, I can see why you're constantly worried about your heart. Your father and uncle suddenly died from heart attacks at your age. But I think we need to look at the facts: Your father and uncle smoked like chimneys and ate nothing but meat and potatoes. You lead a healthy lifestyle. You should listen to your doctors when they say your heart is fine."

2. "*Don't* accuse me of being 'crazy,' 'neurotic,' or a 'faker.' That won't help me get a handle on my anxiety or change it. Instead it creates bad feelings and tension between us."

   Example: Jim's wife had gotten into the habit of blaming him for using his health worries as an excuse for not doing things. This didn't help Jim deal with his anxiety. And it didn't give his wife anything more than a short-lived release of pent-up frustration. After an hour or so she was accusing him of being lazy all over again.

   "Jim, I'm sick of your crazy, lazy excuses. You don't have to take out the trash because of your heart; you don't take the kids to basketball practice because driving is too 'strenuous'; you get to stay home from work and sit in front of the TV all day while I work. I wish you'd just get off your lazy ass and give me some help around here!"

3. "*Do* praise me for the effort I put into learning new ways of coping with my health anxiety. This will help me succeed in breaking my health anxiety cycle. Everybody likes praise and encouragement; it can be enjoyable to give and to receive."

   Examples: There are many different ways of giving praise. It can come in the form of a small token or gesture—a small treat or a hug for a job well done. Carefully chosen words of encouragement are very effective. Here are a few basic ideas, though you'll want to put them in terms that fit your own relationship:

   "Jim, I'm really pleased that lately you haven't been asking me for reassurance. It must be difficult for you at times, but you're doing a great job."

"Aaron, it's great that you've been ignoring your aches and pains and getting on with living. I can't tell you how happy I am to see you out playing golf with your buddies."

"Jessica, I'm really glad that you're ignoring those stomachaches and going to school. And it's really great that you've discovered that the stomach pains disappear when you get involved in something interesting, like your art class."

4. *"Don't* punish me for worrying about my health. Nagging, yelling at me, and threatening me make me feel stressed and, as a result, create the very same bodily sensations that cause me to worry. It makes my health anxiety worse and does nothing good for our relationship."

Examples: Just as praise can come in many forms, so can punishing responses. Here are a few samples of words to avoid using.

"Albert, if you don't stop whining about your sore throat and get to school, I'll give you something to whine about!"

"Honey, you're always bitching about feeling sick. For Christ's sake, why can't you just get over it!"

"Janie, come out of the bathroom this instant! You know that Dr. Taylor said you shouldn't be in there checking the moles on your back. Janie! Are you listening to me?!"

5. *"Do* give yourself a break if you're feeling stressed out with me. It's okay! I understand that my health anxiety is stressful for both of us. You also need your space and time to relax."

Example: Jim's wife felt herself getting frustrated. He'd been working hard at changing the ways he thought about the noise in his body. She'd been helping out but was tired after a long week at work. She realized that getting away for some personal time would be a good thing for everyone.

"Honey, I appreciate that your health anxiety is causing some real problems for you. And I'm glad you're working hard at overcoming it. But I need to take care of *me*, too. So I'm going out shopping for the afternoon with some friends for a while. I'll be back soon."

6. *"Don't* make me feel guilty about my health anxiety. It makes me feel stressed, and this creates the very same bodily sensations that cause me to worry. It doesn't help our relationship, either."

Example: Judy's husband had put up with more of her asking "Do you think I'm okay?" than he could take. He didn't know what to do and just blew up at her. It felt good to get things off his chest, but within a few minutes he was feeling pretty bad about making Judy cry.

"Judy, you're constantly going on and on—and on!—about bowel cancer. Do you realize how stressful that is for *me* to listen to?! Do you think that *I* like hearing about your make-believe diseases?! I just don't know what to do!"

Specific Advice for the Overinvolved Caretaker

Just like our advice to you on helping your stressed-out loved ones to help you, we offer some *dos* and *don'ts* for your overinvolved family and friends to consider. As before, these *dos* and *don'ts* should be considered guidelines rather than rigid rules, and they need to be tried on for size. When you sit down to discuss these things with your family and friends, we can't overemphasize how important it is to let them know that you're not blaming them for your health worries. Be frank in letting them know that you've grown together in such a way that some of the things they do aren't helpful for you in breaking your health anxiety cycle. This, however, isn't their fault or yours. Blame isn't the name of the game, and it won't help anyone. Ask them to think of your health anxiety as a puzzle that you need help to figure out and solve. If you can solve the puzzle of health anxiety together, everyone in your social circle will benefit. But if you (or someone else) place blame, bad feelings will arise.

1. "*Do* understand that I'll have a hard time getting over the idea that there's something seriously wrong with me if you keep fussing over me."

2. "*Don't* blame yourself—or me—for the way your well-intentioned efforts to help have actually been keeping my health anxiety cycle alive. We didn't know this before. Blaming won't help. But now that we know what's helpful and what's not, we can make changes to the things you do for me in a way that will starve my health anxiety."

3. "*Do* try to stop being so protective of me. The doctors have told me my physical health is good, and I'm learning that my worries are largely related to stress and anxiety—things under my control. Although it may be hard for both of us at first, let me start doing things on my own again."

4. "*Don't* support me when I'm worrying and looking for reassurance. Instead of giving me reassurance, which feeds my health anxiety, you could try reinforcing my efforts to change my thoughts and behaviors about disease. And you can reinforce my doctor's message that my physical health is good."

5. "*Do* make sure that there are many important, fulfilling things in your *own* life, aside from caring for me. Make sure to care for yourself! I understand that you need to do this, and I want you to."

Things to Remember

The important message we want to leave you with is that there are several things you can do to help your family and friends to help you overcome your health anxiety. There are some things you can do that will help everyone and others that depend a bit on whether your loved ones are stressed out or overinvolved. Getting people to change their ways is never easy, but, with effort, it can be done. It's pretty likely that you have loved ones who want what's best for you. Get them involved in breaking your health anxiety cycle. Although this is something you can do alone, you'll have greater success with a team effort.

The first step is getting your family and friends to read through the first two chapters of this book so that they have an idea about the nature and causes of health anxiety. Give them some time to digest the information and offer to answer questions they have.

The second step is to sit down with them and openly and nonjudgmentally discuss how your health anxiety affects you *and* how it affects them. Emphasize how reassurance feeds your health anxiety, and use Figure 9 to work out an agreement to kick the reassurance habit. Pick an appropriate time and place for these discussions. We recommend a time when your loved ones aren't rushed or in a hurry to get somewhere. Choose a quiet place that's free from distraction and take the phone off the hook so that you're not interrupted. If need be, have more than one discussion.

Finally, get your loved ones to read through this chapter. They can do this alone or with you present. Because the *dos* and *don'ts* are written as if being presented to them by you, being present will give you an opportunity to give your own examples. You'll also be able to help them identify whether they feel they're in a stressed-out or overinvolved role and assist them in learning how some of the strategies outlined in this chapter can help them help you overcome your health worries. By this point you've become very knowledgeable about health anxiety and are in a good position to help those close to you help you. This is quite an accomplishment!

Where to Turn for Further Help

In the next chapter we discuss professional resources for treating health anxiety. If you decide to see a therapist for additional help with your health anxiety, then consider taking your loved ones so they, too, can meet with the therapist and further discuss things that they can do to help you overcome your health anxiety. If the problem in your relationship is broader than health anxiety, then family or couples therapy might be needed. For example, if you and your partner find that you're having arguments about all sorts of things—finances, child rearing, social activities—then couples counseling might be fruitful. Discuss this with a therapist or doctor.

Ten

Living Life and Maintaining Your Gains

The first nine chapters gave you the tools to break free of the health anxiety cycle and get on with living life. We're hopeful that you've made progress and that you're no longer as worried about your health as you were when you started reading this book. But your practice shouldn't stop here. You should keep practicing until the strategies that work best for you become habitual. This way you'll experience lasting reductions in anxiety. This is what we see in clinical practice. But even after you've taken control of it, everyone experiences times when anxiety flares up. In this chapter we'll give you some pointers on what to do if your health anxiety resurfaces and where to turn if you feel that seeing a health anxiety specialist is right for you. You also need to replace the time you've recaptured from worrying—new free time, so to speak—with things that you enjoy and that make you happy. This will improve your overall sense of well-being, which will also help keep your health anxiety at bay. This chapter shows you a few simple ways you can fill your new free time with activities that enhance your enjoyment of life.

Handling Flare-Ups

Despite having gained control over your health anxiety, you can expect times when it will resurface, and you'll find yourself wondering and maybe even worrying whether the bodily sensations you're experiencing mean you're sick. Sometimes this happens when a lot of stressful things are happening in your life. Other times it can happen when you get sick, when a loved one is struggling with disease, or when there's a media blitz on the "disease of the month." It happens to everyone from time to time. When it happens to you, the best thing to do is to work through the strategies that you found most helpful in conquering your health anxiety the first time around. Most people can take control of health anxiety flare-ups and smother their flames fairly quickly. You have to look at flare-ups for what they are and what they aren't.

They are:

- Common,
- Temporary, short-lived setbacks, and
- Reminders to practice the exercises you've learned to deal with health anxiety (and other stressors in your life).

They are not:

- A sign of relapse or, in other words, that you've lost all the things gained by practicing the strategies in this book, or
- A full-out return of your health anxiety.

The key in taking back control when you do experience a flare-up is remembering that *they are temporary setbacks and not a complete return of health anxiety.* A few specific exercises will help prepare you for quick action against flare-ups.

It's often been said that the best defense is a strong offense. This holds true when the opponent is health anxiety. For this reason we've developed a series of exercises that we call the Health Anxiety Relapse Prevention (HARP) program that will prepare you to be on the offensive when your health anxiety flares up. The HARP program consists of three steps as follows:

1. A review of examples of people who responded to their flare-ups in ways that didn't help,
2. Thinking of ways the people in the examples could have coped better with their flare-ups, and
3. Developing your own personalized HARP program.

Responses That Don't Help

Sometimes people who've overcome their health anxiety will respond to flare-ups in ways that aren't helpful. Most of the time this happens because they forget to use the strategies they learned for breaking their health anxiety cycle in the first place and think that the flare-up is a sign that they're back to square one. Here are a few examples of responses to flare-ups that weren't helpful.

Riley: "That damn program hasn't helped."

Riley had a long history of health anxiety that he'd successfully over-come a few months ago by practicing self-help strategies. But one morn-ing he woke up wheezing. He also had a dry, hacking cough. He started to worry that it could be something serious. "Maybe I have tuberculosis, or it might even be lung cancer," he thought. Soon he had worked him-self up into an extremely anxious state. Riley realized that he'd become very anxious, just as he was before he'd started the self-help program. He thought, "That damn program hasn't helped me a single bit! I'm right back where I started." He didn't use the coping skills he learned and worked so hard at practicing. His health anxiety continued to worsen.

Dory: "I can't even force myself to visit Ken."

Dory had a strong fear of getting cancer. Because of her fear, she'd been staying away from pretty much anything having to do with cancer. She was able to overcome her fear successfully by practicing exposure exer-cises and hadn't been avoiding cancer-related things for almost two years. However, her cancer fear started to return when a close friend was diagnosed with brain cancer. Dory didn't notice that her fear had returned until it was really severe. By that stage she was back to avoid-ing everything that reminded her of cancer. "I can't even force myself to visit Ken, and I know he's probably not going to be around much lon-ger," she'd say to friends. She forgot about the things she'd learned from practicing exposure exercises and felt helpless to deal with the return of her fears.

Helpful Responses

Based on what you've learned from earlier chapters, what could Riley and Dory have done differently in response to the return of their anxiety and fear? Think about this for a few minutes and then answer the questions below.

1. Write down three things that Riley could have done to better cope with his worries about having a respiratory disease. (*Hint*: How might Riley's thoughts influence his health anxiety? Is there any evidence to support his thoughts about tuberculosis or lung cancer? What might he say to himself to feel less anxious? What sorts of things is he doing to make his health anxiety worse? What could he do differently? Does his lapse really mean that his self-help program didn't help "a single bit"?)

- _____
  _____
  _____
  _____

- _____
  _____
  _____
  _____

- _____
  _____
  _____
  _____

2. Write down three things that Dory could have done to better cope with her cancer phobia. (*Hint*: Does avoidance help her in any way? If so, how? If not, why? What things could she do in a step-by-step fashion to overcome her phobia? Should she visit Ken?)

- _____
  _____
  _____
  _____

- _____
  _____
  _____
  _____

- _____
  _____
  _____
  _____

These questions are meant to get you thinking about things you've learned about health anxiety. If you're uncertain of what to write down, look back at some of your worksheets from previous chapters. Look at the examples and illustrations we've provided. You'll find the answers there. Here are a few ideas to get you started.

- Both Riley and Dory viewed their worries and fears as a full-blown return of their health anxiety. They might be able to take back control more quickly if they reinterpret the worry and fear as a temporary, even expected, flare-up.
- Riley immediately jumped to the conclusion that his wheezing and coughing were the result of some disease, perhaps tuberculosis or lung cancer. He could try taking a few minutes to examine the evidence and develop alternate explanations. This would help prevent his anxiety from spiraling out of control.
- Dory wouldn't go visit Ken because she was afraid of catching cancer. Confronting her fear, using exposure exercises to gradually work her way up to visiting Ken, is one thing that would help her cope.

Preparing Your Personalized HARP Program

Your personalized HARP program consists of two parts. The first part involves preparing a plan of response for flare-ups *before* they occur. The second part is a series of steps to work through *when a flare-up actually occurs.*

Part 1: Your Response Plan

Your HARP program response plan is based on the things you've already learned from reading and working through the exercises in this book. Working through the experiences of Riley and Dory should have you thinking about helpful and unhelpful responses to flare-ups. What you'll do now is summarize what you've learned by answering the three following questions. This summary is a list of what *you* should and shouldn't do if you feel your health anxiety returning. Matt (from Chapter 7) completed this exercise, and we've provided his responses in Figure 10, to help you along.

1. Write down all the things you've learned about the *causes* of your health anxiety. You can use extra pages if necessary.

   - _____
   - _____
   - _____
   - _____
   - _____
   - _____
   - _____
   - _____

1. Write down all the things you've learned about the *causes* of your health anxiety. You can use extra pages if necessary.

   - *Focusing on my body makes me notice changes that I think are related to heart disease.*
   - *I used to worry that changes in my heartbeat meant my heart was going to stop. I now know that all kinds of things, like walking up stairs or being under pressure at work, can make my heart beat faster.*
   - *I spend a lot of time looking for information about serious heart disease. This takes away from other things that are important to me and it usually just makes me more anxious.*
   - *I go to my family doctor all of the time hoping that he'll tell me everything is okay. I've even gone to a cardiologist a few times for the same reason.*
   -
   -

2. Write down the things that might help you in the short term but make your health anxiety *worse* in the longer term.

   - *Going to my doctor and the cardiologist for reassurance that I'm not going to drop dead.*
   - *Being inactive. I feel safe when I don't exercise or play with the kids. But I know this isn't good for me in the long run. It's not fair to the kids, either.*
   - *Carrying around my security blanket, my nitroglycerine pills. They make me feel safe, but I understand now that just having them around actually makes me worry about having to use them.*
   -
   -
   -

3. What sorts of things have you learned that help you cope with or even overcome your health anxiety? (*Hint*: These could have to do with using certain exercises to reduce stress [from Chapter 5], the way you think about things [from Chapter 6], or the way you do things [from Chapter 7].)

   - *When I feel stress building up I try to do rapid relaxation. If I have time I take 10 minutes and work through my whole body.*
   - *I know that changes in my heart rate and the way my heart "feels" can be caused by things other than disease. Someday I might have a heart problem. It's possible. When I notice changes, I know I can collect evidence to decide if it's stress, disease, or something else.*
   - *I can also use interoceptive exposure exercises—running on the spot works—to show that a rapidly beating and pounding heart won't harm me.*
   - *I know what exercise I can do if I'm tempted to start carrying my nitro pills again.*
   - *Checking and reassurance seeking are always tempting me. I know that I can examine the evidence for and against the effectiveness of these behaviors in order to remind myself that they're not helpful.*
   -

FIGURE 10. **Matt's completed questions for Part 1 of his HARP program.**

2. Write down the things that might help you in the short term but make your health anxiety *worse* in the longer term.

- _____
- _____
- _____
- _____
- _____
- _____
- _____
- _____

3. What sorts of things have you learned that help you cope with or even overcome your health anxiety? (*Hint*: These could have to do with using certain exercises to reduce stress [from Chapter 5], the way you think about things [from Chapter 6], or the way you do things [from Chapter 7].)

- _____
- _____
- _____
- _____
- _____
- _____
- _____
- _____

Part 2: A Step-by-Step Approach to Flare-Ups

Your answers to part 1 are a reminder of the things you should and shouldn't be doing to keep your health anxiety at bay. Remember, practice turns exercises into habits; in this case, good habits that will keep your health anxiety under control. When a flare-up happens, you need to take back control quickly. Working through the following steps will help you do this.

1. Remind yourself that the flare-up is temporary.

2. Analyze the situation. Try to figure out why the flare-up happened. Write down the frightening thoughts you had during the flare-up, including what you thought might happen. Write down your specific thoughts. *Example*: "My chest pain means I have heart disease."

- _____
- _____
- _____
- _____

3. Review the evidence for and against your frightening thoughts. Are there alternative explanations? Write down alternative explanations. *Example:* "My chest pain is from increased tension in the muscles in my chest, and not from my heart."

- _____
- _____
- _____
- _____

4. Practice the exercises you've learned to change specific thoughts and behaviors related to your health anxiety. Use relaxation and breathing retraining exercises as well. Write down the exercises that you tried in order to get your flare-up under control. Which were most helpful?

- _____
- _____
- _____
- _____

5. Restrict the flare-up. Don't do things that make health anxiety worse— reassurance seeking, checking your body, and avoiding things that frighten you. Write down the things you're trying not to do. *Example:* "I'm not going to give in to my temptation to search the Internet for information about my stomach cramps and diarrhea. And I'm not rushing to the doctor just yet."

- _____
- _____
- _____
- _____

6. Return to any situation that you're starting to avoid. Do this as soon as possible. Develop a step-by-step plan for returning to these situations using the exposure exercises you learned in Chapter 7. If a situation is too anxiety provoking to enter, then try an easier but related situation and

gradually work up to the more difficult situations. List the situations you're avoiding because of fear. List the steps involved in gradually exposing yourself to these situations in order to overcome the fear. *Example*: Dory could begin to overcome her cancer phobia by first looking at magazine articles about cancer survivors and gradually working up to a visit with Ken.

- _____
- _____
- _____
- _____

7. If steps 1 through 6 haven't helped you, then seriously consider contacting someone who specializes in the treatment of the health anxiety disorders. Several professional organizations can help you locate a qualified professional in your area. We've provided a list of these organizations, as well as several therapists from the United States, Canada, and Europe in the Resources section at the back of this book.

Things to Remember

Flare-ups are temporary and short-lived setbacks that can be controlled using the same strategies you used to break your health anxiety cycle. They aren't a full-out return of your health anxiety. The best defense is a well-developed plan of action—your personalized HARP program—to use against flare-ups when they occur. Your HARP program gives you a step-by-step plan that will help you focus on what needs to be done to regain control over your health anxiety. We recommend that you keep a copy of your HARP program in a handy place so that it's available when needed. Keep a copy in your purse or wallet or post it in a place that you're usually near—on your refrigerator, near your computer, on your bathroom mirror. If you're unable to regain control, then seeking treatment from a person who specializes in health anxiety would be worth considering.

Matt: "I'm a new man."

Matt was successful in overcoming his health anxiety and getting back to enjoying quality time with his wife and kids. He did experience two flare-ups in the first six months following completion of his treatment. In each case he worked through his HARP program—which he keeps folded in his wallet to this day—and was able to successfully prevent his anxiety from spiraling out of control. Today Matt's health anxiety has faded into a memory of things past and hasn't been sparked for over three years. He's now helping coach his eldest daughter's baseball team and, inspired by his wife's encouragement and Lance Armstrong's successes, has started doing something he's dreamed of for years—he joined a road cycling club that trains together and tours the countryside every Sunday. In his own words, he's "a new man."

Specialist Treatments for Health Anxiety

When should you think about seeking specialized treatment for your health anxiety? This is a simple question for which there is no easy answer. If you've been suffering with health anxiety for a long time or if you've been unable to break your health anxiety cycle on your own, then you may need specialized treatment to take back control of your life. You might also give serious consideration to getting help from a specialist if:

- Your efforts to break your health anxiety cycle on your own haven't given you the results you desire,
- You're having success with some areas but feel you need coaching with certain aspects of your health-related thoughts and behaviors, or
- You have a flare-up that you're unable to get back under control on your own.

Specialist treatment options for people who have health anxiety are as varied as they are for the other anxiety disorders discussed in Chapter 3. They include medication, hypnosis, approaches based on the teachings of Sigmund Freud, and cognitive-behavioral therapy. Research on health anxiety treatments is in its early stages, but what we do know is increasing quickly. Hypnosis and the Freud-based psychotherapies haven't been shown to be effective with health anxiety; we don't recommend them. The methods for which there is growing evidence of effectiveness include some medications and various components of cognitive-behavioral therapy.

Medication

The SSRI medications Luvox, Paxil, and Prozac have all been studied in people with hypochondriasis. The research shows that people who take an SSRI have greater reductions in symptoms than people not getting any kind of treatment over a period of 8 to 12 weeks. Prozac was found to be the most promising of the medications, giving the greatest overall reduction in symptoms. Unfortunately, little is known about whether the reduction in health anxiety symptoms from taking Prozac is maintained when it's stopped. Prozac may be worth considering and discussing with your doctor if you need immediate relief, if you're unable to devote the time needed for the exercises of self-help and cognitive-behavioral therapy, or if you can't find or don't live near a place where there's a cognitive-behavioral therapist who specializes in the health anxiety disorders.

Cognitive-Behavioral Therapy

Cognitive-behavioral therapy for health anxiety is very similar to the self-help exercises you've been working through in this book. It usually includes some or all of these elements: psychoeducation, stress management, changing ways of thinking about bodily sensations, letting go of unhelpful behaviors, situational and interoceptive exposure, and guidance on active living. Research shows that psychoeducation by itself is very effective in reducing the symptoms of people with moderate levels of health anxiety. This is consistent with our own observations; many of the patients we see feel relief after learning about the health anxiety cycle and the many non-disease-related things that cause their bodily sensations.

A growing number of research studies have shown that various combinations of cognitive-behavioral exercises (or what we call cognitive-behavioral therapy packages) are perhaps the most effective way of treating hypochondriasis. They're at least as effective as taking Prozac, their effects last longer, and they're the first treatment of choice of about three of every four people who seek specialist treatment. The difference between self-help approaches and those used by a cognitive-behavioral therapist is in the degree of coaching and assistance you receive. We've tried to guide you through cognitive-behavioral exercises as best we can without actually being there with you; but you've been on your own in coming up with examples from your own life and in working through any difficult spots that have cropped up during your practice. These are the sorts of things that a cognitive-behavioral therapist with expertise in health anxiety can help you with if need be.

Combined and Sequential Treatment

The merits of combining medication with cognitive-behavioral treatment haven't been researched as of yet. We suspect that a combination of these treatments may work best for people with severe health anxiety. Sequential treatments for health anxiety haven't been researched, either. But the same principles we discussed for the other anxiety disorders apply. We recommend starting with psychoeducation and self-help—the things you've done in working through the exercises in this book—followed by specialized treatment with Prozac or from a cognitive-behavioral therapist as needed to make further gains or regain control after a bad flare-up.

Living Life to Its Fullest

Has your health anxiety caused you to lose touch with many of the activities you once enjoyed or that made you feel good about yourself? Some of the people you met in early chapters had given up a lot—hobbies, favorite sporting activities, playing with their kids, spending quality time with their partners, visiting friends, and making useful contributions at work. Bernard, for example, had abandoned all his favorite pastimes, including playing competitive tennis. He sought treatment for health anxiety and gradually overcame his problems. However, he didn't feel like he was truly living until he returned to his exciting and demanding world of amateur competitive tennis. He enjoyed the blissful fatigue after each match and would often think to himself, "How did I ever let myself get so needlessly worried about my heart? I feel so great after a tough workout on the court."

What did you give up in the past? Things that you really enjoyed but haven't been doing lately? Take a minute to think about these things. List them on the following lines.

1. _____
2. _____
3. _____
4. _____
5. _____
6. _____

Some people find this task easy, but many people have a hard time listing much more than a couple of things. If you had difficulty, it doesn't mean there's no hope. It may simply mean you've been so caught up in the health anxiety cycle that you've lost sight of the enjoyable things in life—a walk in the park, pursuing a hobby, helping the kids with a school project, socializing with friends, listening to music, eating good food, and the like. Completing Worksheet 16 will help you figure out what things you've been doing that bring you pleasure, what things you're not finding fun, and what activities you'd like to be doing but aren't.

To get on with living life, it's important to start adding enjoyable activities to your day-to-day existence. As we've said before, balance in life is very important. Marcy's life used to revolve around checking her blood pressure and going to see doctors. As she became less concerned about her health, she wondered, "Now what? I have all this free time on my hands." Although she continued to take responsible care of her health—she saw her doctor every six months for a review of her mildly elevated blood pressure—she sought to balance her life by engaging in enjoyable activities. She joined a pottery class and soon was

Worksheet 16. *Activities for Enhancing Your Quality of Life*

Instructions: Enjoyable activities are essential to your quality of life. But sometimes people neglect these activities when preoccupied or worried about their health. Look through the following checklist of activities. Did you do any of them in the past week? If so, did you enjoy it? Are there any activities that you haven't done but would like to do? This list might help you think about ways of improving your quality of life.

Activities unrelated to health worries	Indicate (√) which activities you did in the past week.	Were these activities enjoyable? (yes/no)	Indicate (√) which activities you didn't do but would like to do.
Creative activities			
Doing artwork or crafts	_____	_____	_____
Knitting, needlework, sewing	_____	_____	_____
Taking a course in something creative (for example, cooking, photography).	_____	_____	_____
Decorating or redecorating your house or apartment	_____	_____	_____
Woodwork, carpentry, or furniture restoration . . .	_____	_____	_____
Repairing things	_____	_____	_____
Mechanical hobbies (for example, fixing gadgets) .	_____	_____	_____
Photography	_____	_____	_____
Creative writing or doing a journal.	_____	_____	_____
Musical hobbies (for example, singing, dancing, playing an instrument)	_____	_____	_____
Games and entertainment			
Watching TV, videos, or DVDs.	_____	_____	_____
Playing video games	_____	_____	_____
Listening to music or radio programs	_____	_____	_____
Going to the movies.	_____	_____	_____
Going to a play, concert, opera, or ballet	_____	_____	_____
Going to a museum, art gallery, or exhibition . . .	_____	_____	_____
Going to a sporting event	_____	_____	_____
Educational activities that *do not* have to do with gathering information about health and disease			
Reading books, magazines, or newspapers	_____	_____	_____
Going to a lecture on a topic that interests you . .	_____	_____	_____
Learning a foreign language	_____	_____	_____
Surfing the Internet	_____	_____	_____
Learning about computers (for example, learning to make a Web page)	_____	_____	_____
Going to the library	_____	_____	_____

(cont.)

Worksheet 16. Activities for Enhancing Your Quality of Life (cont.)

	Did do:	Enjoyable?	Want to do:
Physical activities			
Playing tennis, squash, or racquetball	_____	_____	_____
Playing golf	_____	_____	_____
Ten-pin bowling.	_____	_____	_____
Water activities (for example, swimming, sailing, canoeing)	_____	_____	_____
Walking or hiking	_____	_____	_____
Jogging, aerobics classes, or working out at a fitness center	_____	_____	_____
Snow sports (skiing, skating, snowboarding)	_____	_____	_____
Bike riding	_____	_____	_____
Horseback riding	_____	_____	_____
Playing team sports (for example, volleyball, hockey, basketball)	_____	_____	_____
Fishing or hunting.	_____	_____	_____
Playing snooker or pool	_____	_____	_____
Social and community activities that *do not* involve discussing health and disease			
Writing, telephoning, or e-mailing friends.	_____	_____	_____
Visiting a friend or inviting a friend to your place	_____	_____	_____
Going out to lunch or dinner with a friend	_____	_____	_____
Giving a party or going to a party	_____	_____	_____
Going on a date	_____	_____	_____
Joining a club (for example, a book club or social club) . .	_____	_____	_____
Going to a bar or restaurant	_____	_____	_____
Involvement in community or political activities	_____	_____	_____
Involvement in religious or church activities.	_____	_____	_____
Other			
Sitting in the sun	_____	_____	_____
Going for a scenic drive	_____	_____	_____
Gardening, caring for houseplants, or arranging flowers . .	_____	_____	_____
Visiting fun or interesting places (for example, park, beach, zoo)	_____	_____	_____
Caring for or being with pets	_____	_____	_____
Planning or going on a vacation.	_____	_____	_____
Going to a sauna	_____	_____	_____
Soaking in the bathtub	_____	_____	_____
Doing yoga or meditation.	_____	_____	_____
Buying yourself something special.	_____	_____	_____
Hobbies (for example, stamp collecting, model building, flying a kite)	_____	_____	_____
List your favorite activities here, if they are not listed above:			
_____	_____	_____	_____
_____	_____	_____	_____
_____	_____	_____	_____

Source: Adapted from S. Taylor and G. J. G. Asmundson (2004). *Treating health anxiety: A cognitive-behavioral approach*. New York: Guilford Press. Adapted by permission.

absorbed with ceramics. Instead of constantly worrying about her health, she was now having fun. She felt that her life was in balance; she was looking after the serious matters, keeping her blood pressure in check, but also taking time for fun. As a result she also became less tense, and her blood pressure returned to normal.

If you identified activities on Worksheet 16 that you've been doing but aren't enjoying, replace them with something you'd get more pleasure from. If you're doing some things that are fun, continue doing them. Keep a record of what you do for fun over the next three weeks and rate how enjoyable you find each activity. Set aside some dedicated time for these activities. Use the time-management strategies from Chapter 5 and make a wholehearted effort to do them without letting distractions get in the way. Worksheet 17 can be used to keep track of your activities and ratings of them. Make your ratings using a 5-point scale with 0 indicating *no enjoyment* and 4 indicating *a lot of enjoyment*. Activities that you find to be so-so would be rated at 2. At the end of each week, take a look at your ratings. Keep doing the things that have ratings that are 3 or 4 on average and replace the ones that are usually lower than 3 with something else. It'll take some trial and error, but eventually you'll come up with a list of things that bring you true enjoyment.

Karen enjoyed walking her dog along the meandering trials that skirted the lakeside of the neighborhood park. When working through Worksheet 16 she realized that, despite enjoying these walks, she had not been to the park for years. This was something she definitely wanted to get back to doing on a regular basis. She also decided to start taking in a movie every week with friends. Karen rated her enjoyment of walking in the park and going to the movies with friends for a three-week period. The walks were a big hit, with her ratings averaging a solid 4. The movies, on the other hand, came in at 2 on the 0-to-4 scale. She kept walking and stopped going to the movies. Still wanting to spend time with friends, she tried dinner parties, poker nights, and coffee dates. The dinner parties and coffee dates rated highly, and today Karen and three other friends take turns hosting a monthly gourmet dinner. All in all Karen tested her enjoyment of eight different activities and found three—walks in the park, dinner parties, and coffee dates—that she now does on a regular basis.

In addition to scheduling time for pleasurable activities, you can do other things to improve your overall quality of life. We recommend that you continue using the relaxation and breathing retraining exercises from Chapter 5 to reduce the stress of daily life. And try to do the things that we should all be doing to maximize our sense of well-being—exercise regularly, eat a balanced diet, get six to eight hours of sleep most nights, and smoke or drink only in moderation. Changing your health habits can be a challenge. But, having succeeded in breaking your health anxiety cycle, you've developed skills that will help you work through the challenges of pursuing a healthier lifestyle. This can directly reduce your health anxiety—a program of physical exercise can prove to you

Worksheet 17. Activity Enjoyment Rating Form

Instructions: List each activity you do for enjoyment over the next few weeks. Rate the enjoyment the activity brings you using a scale with 0 = no enjoyment and 4 = a lot of enjoyment.

Day and date	Activity	Enjoyment rating
Example	Went to a movie	3
Example	Took my kids to play in the park	4

that you're not frail and ready to keel over at any minute. We want you to live an enjoyable life free of unnecessary stress and turmoil. You've worked hard at taking back the control over your life that had been wrested away by health anxiety. Now you deserve to enjoy it!

A Final Word

We started this book by having you ask yourself the question "Do I worry too much about my health?" We asked you a number of other questions, as well, and had you complete a paper-and-pencil test called the Whiteley Index. The main reason for beginning this way was to get you thinking—about how your worries about health and disease affect your life and about whether the strategies that we had to offer might be worth trying.

If you're reading this sentence, we know one of two things to be true— you've either tried working through the exercises we laid out for you *or* you're thinking about doing so but wanted to read the whole book first. Either way, excellent! You should be very proud of yourself for making a wholehearted effort to understand your health anxiety and take back control of your life. It's our sincere hope that you've been able to (or will) use what you learned from reading this book to successfully break your health anxiety cycle and that you can continue to keep it at bay. Flare-ups will occur. Remember that they happen to everyone from time to time and that you can use your personalized HARP program to deal with them. If you're having difficulties with certain aspects of your health anxiety—some nagging thought or behavior that you can't kick on your own—think about seeing a health anxiety specialist. A specialist can also help if you have a flare-up that can't be brought under control or if, despite your courageous efforts, you're unable to overcome your worries using self-help.

We'll finish the book in the same way we began—by asking you a few questions. Do you spend a big chunk of each day worrying about the causes of your bodily sensations, checking your body for changes, surfing the Internet for information about certain diseases, or seeking reassurance from others that you're okay? Are you afraid your body is suffering a malfunction or breakdown? Do friends and family tell you that you worry too much or call you a hypochondriac or germ phobic? Do you continue to visit the doctor every time your body gets noisy? Is your score on the Whiteley Index 8 or higher? The ancient Greek philosopher Aristotle said that we are what we do every day. If you've been working at dealing with health anxiety on a daily basis, it's very likely your answers to these questions have changed from the ones you gave when you first started reading this book. It's also very likely that you are now or will soon be well *without worry!*

Resources

Audio and Video

Asmundson, G. J. H. Health anxiety podcast with the Anxiety Disorders Association of America. *http://www.adaa.org/resources-professionals/podcasts/health-anxiety*

Ross, J. (2001). *Freedom from anxiety.* Chicago: Nightingale-Conant. Available from *www.rosscenter.com.* This is a self-help version of a program offered at the Ross Center for Anxiety and Related Disorders in Washington, D.C. It is not specific to health anxiety but may be useful to people with disease phobia.

Additional Books

Abramowitz, J. S., & Braddock, A. E. (2009). *Psychological treatment of health anxiety and hypochondriasis: A biopsychosocial approach.* Cambridge: Hogrefe Publishing.

Antony, M. M., & Norton, P. J. (2009). *The anti-anxiety workbook: Proven strategies to overcome worry, phobias, pain, and obsessions.* New York: Guilford Press.

Asmundson, G. J. G., Taylor, S., & Cox, B. J. (Eds.). (2001). *Health anxiety: Clinical and research perspectives on hypochondriasis and related disorders.* Chichester, UK: Wiley.

Barsky, A. J. (1988). *Worried sick: Our troubled quest for wellness.* Boston: Little, Brown.

Barsky, A. J., & Deans, E. C. (2006). *Stop being your symptoms and start being yourself: The 6-week mind-body program to ease your chronic symptoms.* New York: William Morrow.

Bourne, E. J. (2000). *The anxiety and phobia workbook* (3rd ed.). Oakland, CA: New Harbinger.

Cantor, C. (1996). *Phantom illness: Shattering the myth of hypochondria.* Boston: Houghton Mifflin.

Furer, P., Walker, J. R., & Stein, M. B. (2007). *Treating health anxiety and fear of death: A practitioner's guide.* New York: Springer.

Greenberger, D., & Padesky, C. A. (1995). *Mind over mood: Change how you feel by changing the way you think.* New York: Guilford Press.

Leahy, R. L. (2005). *The worry cure: Seven steps to stop worry from stopping you.* New York: Harmony Books.

Owens, K., & Antony, M. (2011). *Overcoming health anxiety: Letting go of your fear of illness.* Oakland, CA: New Harbinger.

Ross, J. (1995). *Triumph over fear: A book of help for people with anxiety, panic, and phobias.* New York: Bantam Doubleday Dell.

Starcevic, V., & Lipsitt, D. R. (Eds.). (2001). *Hypochondriasis: Modern perspectives on an ancient malady.* New York: Oxford University Press.

Taylor, S., & Asmundson, G. J. G. (2004). *Treating health anxiety: A cognitive behavioral approach.* New York: Guilford Press.

Welch, G. H. (2004). *Should I be tested for cancer?: Maybe not and here's why.* Berkeley: University of California Press.

Wilson, R., & Veale, D. (2009). *Overcoming health anxiety: A self-help guide using cognitive behavioral techniques.* London: Constable and Robinson.

Zgourides, G. D. (2008). *Stop worrying about your health!: How to quit obsessing about symptoms and feel better now.* Lulu.com.

For Children

Quigley, J. (1997). *Johnny germ head.* New York: Holt.

Websites

There are a number of websites that are potential sources of valuable information or support. We recommend that you visit these sites *only* if you want to gather specific information about potential treatment providers. We discourage you from searching these sites for information about disease. We are not responsible for the content or quality of the information that these websites provide.

National Organizations

www.psych.org
www.apa.org
www.adaa.org
www.cacbt.ca
www.cpa.ca
www.nimh.nih.gov
www.bps.org.uk

Cognitive-Behavioral Therapists
with Expertise in Treating Health Anxiety

The following is a list of therapists who have identified themselves, from professional associations, as having expertise in treating health anxiety. The list is not exhaustive; there are many other practitioners with expertise in treating health anxiety who are not included in this list. Even so, this list may be helpful if you are searching for a therapist near you.

United States

California

Mudita Bahadur, PhD, 1137 2nd Street, Suite 213, Santa Monica, CA 90403; Tel.: 310-463-7913; E-mail: *mudita.bahadur@gmail.com*

Hugh Baras, PhD, 415 Cambridge Avenue, Suite 14, Palo Alto, CA 94306; Tel.: 650-325-9002; E-mail: *baras@bigfoot.com*

Rodney Boone, PhD, UCLA Anxiety Disorders Program, UCLA School of Medicine, Department of

Psychiatry, 24445 Hawthorne Boulevard, Suite 105, Torrance, CA 90505; Tel.: 310-375-4855; E-mail: *rpboone@ucla.edu*

Simone K. Madan, PhD, University of California, San Francisco/Mt. Zion General Medicine Clinic, 1701 Divisadero Street, Suite 500, San Francisco, CA 94115; E-mail: *Simone.Madan@ ucsfmedctr.org*

Emanuel Maidenberg, PhD, Neuropsychiatric Institute, UCLA; Tel.: 310-794-1474; E-mail: *emaidenberg@mednet.ucla.edu*

Jacqueline B. Persons, PhD, Joan Davidson, PhD, and Michael A. Tompkins, PhD, San Francisco Bay Area Center for Cognitive Therapy, 5435 College Avenue, Suite 108, Oakland, CA 94618-1598; Tel.: 510-652-4455, ext. 12; E-mail: *mat@sfbacct.com*; Website: *www.sfbacct.com*

David Plotkin, PhD, (*offices in West Los Angeles and Encino*): West Los Angeles, CA: 1964 Westwood Boulevard, Suite 310, Los Angeles, CA 90025; Tel.: 310-285-8355, ext. 20; E-mail: *drplotkin@ gmail.com*; Website: *www.davidplotkinphd.com*

Gerald Tarlow, PhD, 2730 Wilshire Boulevard, Suite 600, Santa Monica, CA 90403; Tel.: 310-208-4077

Colorado

Pamela Brody, PhD, Cognitive Behavior Associates of Denver, 600 South Cherry Street, Suite 725, Denver, CO 80246; Tel.: 303-482-1114; Website: *www.cbtdenver.com*

Connecticut

David F. Tolin, PhD, Director, Anxiety Disorders Center, The Institute of Living, Yale University School of Medicine, 200 Retreat Avenue, Hartford, CT 06106; Tel.: 860-545-7685; Website: *www.instituteofliving.org/adc/index.htm*

Florida

Robert Heller, EdD, Boca Raton, FL; Tel.: 561-451-2731; E-mail: *rheller2007@comcast.net*; Website: *www.robertheller.net*

Georgia

Charles Melville, PhD, 25-B Lenox Pointe, Atlanta, GA 30324; Tel.: 404-266-8881; E-mail: *CHMelville@comcast.net*; Website: *www.drcharlesmelville.com*

Illinois

Mona H. Berman, MA, LCPC, 550 Frontage Road, Suite 2424, Northfield, IL 60093; Tel.: 847-604-1848

John E. Calamari, PhD, Department of Psychology, Finch University of Health Sciences/The Chicago Medical School, 3333 Green Bay Road, North Chicago, IL 60064; Tel.: 847-578-8747; E-mail: *John.Calamari@finchcms.edu*

David Carbonell, PhD, 155 North Michigan Avenue, Suite 528, Chicago, IL 60601; Tel.: 847-481-5251; Website: *www.anxietycoach.com*

James Dod, PhD, 1200 Shermer Road, Suite 208, Northbrook, IL 60062; Tel.: 847-480-1341; E-mail: *jdod@SimplePsychology.com*

Ira S. Halper, MD, Cognitive Therapy Center, 1725 W. Harrison Street, Suite 958, Chicago, IL 60612; Tel.: 312-226-0300; E-mail: *ira_halper@rush.edu*; Website: *www.IraHalper.YourMD.com*

Seoka Salstrom, PhD, Anxiety and Agoraphobia Treatment Center, 1500 Skokie Boulevard, Suite 204, Northbrook, IL 60062; Tel.: 847-559-0001, ext. 6

Joseph R. Zander, PhD, Advocate Medical Group, Department of Psychiatry, 1875 West Dempster Street, Suite 470, Park Ridge, IL 60068; Tel.: 847-723-5865

Rick Zinbarg, PhD, Department of Psychology, Northwestern University, 2029 Sheridan Road, Swift Hall 302, Evanston, IL 60208-0828; Tel.: 847-902-9703; E-mail: *rzinbarg@northwestern.edu*

Maine

James Claiborn, PhD, 6 D Street, South Portland, ME 04106; Tel.: 207-799-0408; E-mail: *anxietyshrink@myfairpoint.net*

Massachusetts

Arthur Barsky, MD, Department of Psychiatry, Brigham and Women's Hospital and Harvard Medical School, 75 Francis Street, Boston, MA 02115; E-mail: *abarsky@partners.org*

Daniel Beck, LICSW, School of Public Health, Health and Social Behavior Research Unit, 1637 Tremont Street, Boston, MA 02120; Tel.: 617-470-3900; E-mail: *dtbck@aol.com*

Jennifer D. Lish, PhD, Worcester Center for Cognitive Behavior Therapy, 9 Cedar Street, Worcester, MA 01609; Tel.: 508-210-0114; E-mail: *jenniferlish@charter.net*

Laurie Livingston, EdD, 1131 Beacon Street, Suite 1, Brookline, MA 02446; Tel.: 617-734-5779; E-mail: *laurie.livingston@comcast.net*

Sabine Wilhelm, PhD, OCD Spectrum Disorders Clinic, Massachusetts General Hospital, Building 149, 13th Street, Charlestown, MA 02129; Tel.: 617-726-6766; E-mail: *sabinewilhelm@ earthlink.net*

Missouri

C. Alec Pollard, PhD, Director, Anxiety Disorders Center, Saint Louis Behavioral Medicine Institute, Saint Louis University, 1129 Macklind Avenue, St. Louis, MO 63110; Tel.: 314-534-0200, ext. 424; E-mail: *info@slbmi.com*; Website: *www.slbmi.com*

New Jersey

Carol J. Dorfman, PhD, 155 North Dean Street, 3rd floor, Englewood, NJ 07631; (*Clinics in Englewood and Livingston*); Tel.: 201-569-4422; E-mail: *drcaroldorfman@gmail.com*; Website: *http://therapists.psychologytoday.com/rms/57701*

Steven B. Gordon, PhD, Director, Behavior Therapy Associates, P.A., 35 Clyde Road, Suite 101, Somerset, NJ 08873; Tel.: 732-873-1212; E-mail: *Btapc@aol.com*; Website: *www.behaviortherapyassociates.com*

James Korman, PsyD, 1474 Route 23 North, Suite 6, Wayne, NJ 07470; (*Clinics in Wayne and Berkeley Heights*); Tel.: 973-694-2022

Sue Schonberg, PhD, Cognitive Therapy and Consultation, 35 DeForest Avenue, Summit, NJ 07901; Tel.: 908-273-3133

Nivine T. Shenouda, PhD, 85 Hopper Avenue, Suite 9, Waldwick, NJ 07463; Tel.: 201-444-9114

New Mexico

Charles H. Elliott, PhD, 3615 N.M. Highway 528, Suite 200, Albuquerque, NM 87114; E-mail: *celliott@psychauthors.com*

New York

Cindy J. Aaronson, PhD, 740 West End Avenue, Suite 5A, New York, NY 10025; (*Clinics in New York and White Plains*); Tel.: 914-472-7398; E-mail: *cindy.aaronson@mssm.edu*

Rochelle Balter, PhD, 228 East 52nd Street, Office A, New York, NY 10022; E-mail: *rbalt@aol.com*

Oshra Cohen, PhD, 441 Route 306, Suite 302, Monsey, NY 10952; Tel.: 305-851-5637

Yoav Cohen, PhD, 286 Madison Avenue, PH, New York, NY 10017; Tel.: 347-831-0280; E-mail: *mail@dryoavcohen.com*; Website: *www.dryoavcohen.com*

Carol L. Friedland, PhD, Ten East End Avenue, Suite 1N, New York, NY 10075; Tel.: 212-585-2700; E-mail: *drcfriedland@gmail.com*

Daniel Gomez, LCSW, 280 Madison Avenue (at 40th Street), New York, NY 10016; Tel.: 917-817-6008; E-mail: *CTLCSW@msn.com*; Website: *www.DanielGomezLcsw.com*

Paul Greene, PhD, Manhattan Center for Cognitive-Behavior Therapy, 276 Fifth Avenue, Suite 905, New York, NY 10001; Tel.: 917-693-6186; E-mail: *dr.paul.greene@gmail.com*; Website: *www.drpaulgreene.com*

Stephen Josephson, PhD, 815 Fifth Avenue, New York, NY 10065; Tel.: 212-888-2777

Jonathan Kaplan, PhD, 105 East 15th Street, #6, New York, NY 10003; Tel.: 888-343-6031; E-mail: *doctor@jonathanskaplan.com*; Website: *www.jonathanskaplan.com*

Jeffrey Kassinove, PhD, 175 West 79th Street, Suite 1A, New York, NY 10024; Tel.: 212-479-7361, ext. 4; (*Clinics in New York and Merrick*); Website: *www.nypsychological.com*

Jeffrey M. Lackner, PhD, Behavioral Medicine Clinic, Department of Medicine, University of Buffalo, School of Medicine, SUNY, ECMC, 462 Grider Street, Buffalo, NY 14215; Tel.: 716-898-5671

Robert L. Leahy, PhD, Director, American Institute for Cognitive Therapy, 136 East 57th Street, Suite 1101, New York, NY 10022; Tel.: 212-308-2440; E-mail: *Leahy@CognitiveTherapyNYC.com*; Website: *www.cognitivetherapynyc.com*

Michael Maher, PhD, 110 East 40th Street, New York, NY 10016; Tel.: 917-226-3774

Dean McKay, PhD, Institute for Cognitive Behavior Therapy and Research, 333 Westchester Avenue, White Plains, NY 10604; Tel.: 914-428-4745

Michael McKee, PhD, 45 Popham Road, Suite 1H, Scarsdale, NY 10583; Tel.: 914-584-9352; Website: *www.MichaelMcKeePhD.com*

Deborah K. Melamed, PhD, SohoCognitive, 560 Broadway, Suite 510, New York, NY 10012; Tel.: 212-925-9833; E-mail: *dmelamed@SohoCognitive.com*; Website: *www.SohoCognitive.com*

Peregrine Murphy Kavros, PhD, 4 West 109th Street, Suite 2D, New York, NY 10025; Tel.: 914-420-6448; E-mail: *drkavros@attention-cbt.com*; Website: *www.attention-cbt.com*

Fugen Neziroglu, PhD, Bio-Behavioral Institute; 925 Northern Boulevard, Great Neck, NY 11021; Tel.: 516-487-7116; E-mail: *Neziroglu@aol.com*; Website: *www.bio-behavioral.com*

Wendy R. Penzel, PsyD and Fred Penzel, PhD, 755 New York Avenue, Suite 200, Huntington, NY 11743; Tel.: 631-673-1225 or 631-351-1729

Simon A. Rego, PsyD, ABPP, ACT, Montefiore Medical Center, Department of Psychiatry and Behavioral Sciences, 111 East 210th Street, Bronx, NY 10467; E-mail: *srego@montefiore.org*; Website: *www.simonrego.com*

Constance J. Salhany, PhD, Cognitive Therapy of Staten Island, 1110 South Avenue @ Lois Lane, Suite 5, Staten Island, NY 10314; Tel.: 347-273-1290; E-mail: *info@cognitivetherapysi.com*; Website: *www.cognitivetherapysi.com*

John Silvestre, MS, LCSW, Cognitive Behavioral Psychotherapy, 680 West End Avenue, Suite 1B, New York, NY 10025; Tel.: 212-362-5413; 2 Blueberry Hill Road, Irvington, NY 10533; Tel.: 914-830-7923; E-mail: *jsilves836@aol.com*; Website: *www.johnsilvestre.com*

Mark Sisti, PhD, ACT, Suffolk Cognitive-Behavioral, 7504 Sixth Avenue, Brooklyn, NY 11209; (*Clinics in Brooklyn, Huntington, and South Setauket*); Tel.: 631-696-2896; Website: *www.suffolkcognitivetherapy.com*

North Carolina

Jonathan S. Abramowitz, PhD, Department of Psychology, University of North Carolina at Chapel Hill, Davie Hall, Campus Box 3270, Chapel Hill, NC 27599; Tel.: 919-843-8170; E-mail: *jabramowitz@unc.edu*

R. Trent Codd, III, EdS, Cognitive-Behavioral Therapy Center of Western North Carolina, 417 Biltmore Avenue, Suite 2E, Asheville, NC 28801; Tel.: 828-350-1177; E-mail: *rtcodd@behaviortherapist.com*; Website: *www.BehaviorTherapist.com*

Reid Wilson, PhD, Anxiety Disorders Treatment Center, 421 Bennett Orchard Trail, Chapel Hill, NC 27516; Tel.: 919-942-0700; E-mail: *rrw@med.unc.edu*; Website: *www.anxieties.com*

Oklahoma

Kim A. Coon, EdD, Department of Psychiatry, The University of Oklahoma College of Medicine, Tulsa, 4502 East 41st Street, Tulsa, OK 74135; Tel.: 918-660-3511; E-mail: *kim-coon@ouhsc.edu*

Pennsylvania

Judith S. Beck, PhD and Norman D. Cotterell, PhD, Beck Institute for Cognitive Therapy and Research, One Belmont Avenue, Suite 700, Bala Cynwyd, PA 19004; Tel.: 610-664-3020

Frank M. Dattilio, PhD, Department of Psychiatry, Harvard Medical School, 1251 S. Cedar Crest Boulevard, Suite 304D, Allentown, PA 18103; Tel.: 610-434-6960; E-mail: *frankdattilio@cs.com*; Website: *www.dattilio.com*

Robert H. Kuehnel, PhD, The Wynnewood House, Suite 207, 300 East Lancaster Avenue, Wynnewood, PA 19096-2142; Tel.: 610-291-0105; E-mail: *rkuehnel@mail.med.upenn.edu*

Chris Molnar, PhD, Mindful Exposure Therapy for Anxiety (META) and Psychological Wellness Center, 1800 Horace Avenue, Abington, PA 19001; Tel.: 267-287-8347; E-mail: *chris@molnarpsychology.com*; Website: *www.meta4stress.com*

Kristin Tatrow, PhD, Advanced Counseling Services, 3895 Adler Place, Suite 130A, Bethlehem, PA 18017; (*Clinics in Bethlehem and Jenkintown*); Tel.: 610-457-0380; Website: *www.doctortatrow.com*

Tennessee

Denise D. Davis, PhD, Clinical Psychologist, 108 Harding Place, Suite 201, Nashville, TN 37205; Tel.: 615-356-5075; Website: *www.denisedavisphd.com*

Texas

Saharah Shrout, Program Manager, The Houston OCD Program, 1401 Castle Court, Houston, TX 77006; Tel.: 713-526-5055; E-mail: *info@houstonOCDprogram.org*; Website: *www.HoustonOCDprogram.org*

Virginia

Albert Jerome, PhD, Ashburn Psychological Services, 44110 Ashburn Shopping Plaza, Suite 251, Ashburn, VA 20147; Tel.: 703-723-2999; E-mail: *DrAl@draljerome.com*; Website: *www.draljerome.com*

Washington State

James A. Keyes, PhD, Group Health, 1730 Minor Avenue, #1400, Seattle, WA 98101; Tel.: 206-287-2500

David J. Kosins, PhD, 318 W. Galer Street, Suite 201, Seattle, WA 98119; Tel.: 206-285-0900; E-mail: *dkosins@u.washington.edu*; Website: *www.davidkosins.com*

Stephen Sholl, EdD, 2200 24th Avenue East, Seattle, WA 98112; Tel.: 206-328-0910; E-mail: *StephenSholl@aol.com*

Wisconsin

Gregory G. Kolden, PhD, University of Wisconsin, Department of Psychiatry, 6001 Research Park Boulevard, Madison, WI 53719-1179; Tel.: 608-263-6082; E-mail: *ggkolden@wisc.edu*

Bradley C. Riemann, PhD, Director, OCD Center and Cognitive Behavioral Therapy Services, Rogers Memorial Hospital, 34700 Valley Road, Oconomowoc, WI 53066; Tel.: 800-767-4411, ext. 1388

Australia

Christopher Mogan, PhD, The Anxiety Clinic, Melbourne Clinic Consulting Suites, Suite 6/140 Church Street, Richmond, Victoria 3121, Australia; E-mail: *mogan@theanxietyclinic.com*; Website: *www.theanxietyclinic.com/index.html*

Canada

Alberta

Kerry Mothersill, PhD, 609 14th Street NW, Room 509, Calgary, Alberta, T2N 2A1; Tel.: 403-571-1781; E-mail: *kerry.mothersill@albertahealthservices.ca*

British Columbia

North Shore Stress and Anxiety Clinic, 145 Chadwick Court, Suite 330, Lonsdale Quay, North Vancouver, British Columbia, V7M 3K1; Tel.: 604-985-3535; Toll free: 1-866-985-3535; Website: *www.nssac.ca/index.html*

Steven Welch, PhD, 1480 Foster Street, Suite 26, White Rock, British Columbia, V4B 3X7; Tel.: 604-535-3393 (ext. 2)

Maureen Whittal, PhD, Vancouver CBT Centre, Suite 708-777 West Broadway, Vancouver, British Columbia; Tel.: 604-738-7337; E-mail: *maureen.whittal@vancouvercbt.ca*; Website: *www.vancouvercbt.ca*

Manitoba

John Walker, PhD and Patricia Furer, PhD, Anxiety Disorders Program, M5—St. Boniface General Hospital, 409 Tache Avenue, Winnipeg, Manitoba, R2H 2A6; Tel.: 204-237-2055; E-mail: *jwalker@sbgh.mb.ca*

New Brunswick

David A. Clark, PhD, 72 Lansdowne Street, Fredericton, New Brunswick, E3B 1T2; Tel.: 506-459-8315; E-mail: *clark@unb.ca*

Nova Scotia

Sherry Stewart, PhD, Fenwick Psychological Services, Fenwick Medical Centre, 5595 Fenwick Street, Suite 314, Halifax, Nova Scotia, B3H 4M2; Tel.: 902-421-7514; E-mail: *sstewart@dal.ca*

Ontario

Martin M. Antony, PhD, Director, Anxiety Treatment and Research Centre, St. Joseph's Healthcare, Hamilton, Fontbonne Building, 6th floor, 50 Charlton Avenue East, Hamilton, Ontario, L8N 4A6; Tel.: 905-522-1155, ext. 33048; E-mail: *mantony@stjoes.ca*; Website: *www.anxietytreatment.ca*

Anxiety Disorders Clinic, McMaster University Medical Centre, Hamilton Health Sciences, 1200 Main Street West, Hamilton, Ontario, L8N 3Z5; Tel.: 905-521-2100, ext. 76181; Fax: 905-521-2628; E-mail: *vanamer@mcmaster.ca*

Eilenna Denisoff, PhD and Peter Farvolden, PhD, CBT Associates of Toronto, 100 Adelaide Street West, Toronto, Ontario, M5H 1S3; Tel.: 416-363-4228; E-mail: *drdenisoff@cbtassociates.net*

Trevor Hart, PhD, 114 Maitland Street, Toronto, Ontario, M4Y 1E1; Tel.: 416-979-5000, ext. 6192; E-mail: *therapy@drhart.ca*

Margret Hovanec, PhD, Massey College, 4 Devonshire Place, Toronto, Ontario, M5S 2E1; Tel.: 416-861-1562; E-mail: *mhovanec@sympatico.ca*

Martin Katzman, MD, START Clinic for the Mood and Anxiety Disorders, 32 Park Road, Toronto, Ontario, M4W 2N4; Tel.: 416-598-9344; E-mail: *mkatzman@startclinic.ca*; Website: *www.startclinic.ca*

David A. Moscovitch, PhD, Department of Psychology, University of Waterloo, 200 University Avenue West, Waterloo, Ontario, N2L 3G1; Tel.: 519-888-4567, ext. 32549; E-mail: *dmosco@uwaterloo.ca*

Neil Pilkington, PhD, 2 Carlton Street, Suite 1718, Toronto, Ontario, M5B 1J3; Tel.: 416-977-5666; E-mail: *dr.neil.pilkington@rogers.com*

Quebec

Adam S. Radomsky, PhD, Department of Psychology, Concordia University, 7141 Sherbrooke Street West, Montreal, Quebec, H4B 1R6; Tel.: 514-848-2424, ext. 4579; E-mail: *Adam.Radomsky@concordia.ca*

Debbie Sookman, PhD, Department of Psychology, McGill University Health Centre and Training Director, 1025 Pine Avenue West, Montreal, Quebec, H3A 1A1; Tel.: 514-842-1231, ext. 34290; E-mail: *Debbie.Sookman@mcgill.ca*

Saskatchewan

Heather Hadjistavropoulos, PhD, Department of Psychology, University of Regina, Regina, Saskatchewan, S4S 0A2; Tel.: 306-585-5133; Website: *www.uregina.ca/arts/psychology/faculty/hadj-h.htm*

Colombia

Luis Eduardo Peña, Clínica Farallones, Calle 9C #5-25, Consultorio 804, Cali, Colombia; Tel.: +572-487-8084; E-mail: *luispena@misicologo.com*; Website: *www.misicologo.com*

France

Pierre Lamy, MPs, Centre médical La Villanelle, Route de Toulouse, 31700 Cornebarrieu, France; Tel.: 05-34-52-94-19; E-mail: *pierrelamy52@orange.fr*

Iceland

The Icelandic Center for Treatment of Anxiety Disorders, 104 Reykjavik, Iceland; Tel.: 011-354-534-0110 or 011-354822-0043; E-mail: *kms@kms.is*; Website: *www.kms.is*

The Netherlands

Theo K. Bouman, PhD, Department of Clinical Psychology, University of Groningen, Grote Kruisstraat 2, 9712 TS Groningen, The Netherlands; E-mail: *t.k.bouman@rug.nl*

Paul M. G. Emmelkamp, PhD, Oosterpark 81, 1092 AV Amsterdam; E-mail: *P.M.G.Emmelkamp@ uva.nl*

Norway

Ingvard Wilhelmsen, Department of Medicine, Haraldsplass Deaconal Hospital, University of Bergen, N-5009 Bergen; Tel.: 47-55-979-427; E-mail: *Ingvard.wilhelmsen@med.uib.no*

Sweden

Magnus Adell, Leg psykolog, Kungsängsgatan 5B, 757 52 Uppsala, Sweden; Tel.: 070-417-6706; E-mail: *magnus.adell@telia.com*

Eva Frykman, MD, Vallentinhuset, Sabbatsbergsvägen 8, S-112 61 Stockholm, Sweden; Tel.: 46-708-309976; E-mail: *eva.frykman@vallentinhuset.se*

Lisa Grönblad, Leg psycholog, Stockholms KBT-praktik, Götgatan 71, 116 21 Stockholm, Sweden; Tel.: 46-8-5000-3721; E-mail: *lisa.gronblad@stockholmskbt.se*; Website: *www.stockholmskbt.se*

Amanda Hicks, Leg psycholog, Vasagatan, Tranås, Sweden; Tel.: 076-336-7890 and 070-575-4975; Website: *www.kbtcentralen.com*

Carema Hjärnhälsan (Clinic), Nacka, Stockholm, Sweden; *(Clinics in Nacka, Värmdö, Tyresö, Haninge, and Nynäshamn)*; Tel.: 46-8-718-7190

Lena Dur Högnelid, Leg psycholog, KBT blå dur, Usedomsvägen 10, 120 47 Enskede gård, Sweden; Tel.: 46-0-709-508-532; E-mail: *info@kbtbladur.se*; Website: *www.kbtbladur.se*

Dan Katz, Leg psykolog, Katz KBT-konsult AB (private practice); Västerlånggatan 27, 111 29 Stockholm, Sweden; Tel.: 46-0-708-360-883; E-mail: *dan.katz@katzkbt.se*

Björn Paxling, Leg psycholog, Storgatan 41, 211 42 Malmö, Sweden; Tel.: 46-733-720-229; E-mail: *bjorn.paxling@gmail.com*

Worksheets

The Whiteley Index

Here are some questions about your health. Circle either YES or NO to indicate your answer to each question.

1. Do you often worry about the possibility that you have got a serious illness? YES NO

2. Are you bothered by many pains and aches? YES NO

3. Do you find that you are often aware of various things happening in your body? YES NO

4. Do you worry a lot about your health? YES NO

5. Do you often have the symptoms of very serious illness? YES NO

6. If a disease is brought to your attention (through the radio, television, newspapers, or someone you know) do you worry about getting it yourself? YES NO

7. If you feel ill and someone tells you that you are looking better, do you become annoyed? YES NO

8. Do you find that you are bothered by many different symptoms? YES NO

9. Is it easy for you to forget about yourself, and think about all sorts of other things? YES NO

10. Is it hard for you to believe the doctor when he or she tells you there is nothing for you to worry about? YES NO

11. Do you get the feeling that people are not taking your illness seriously enough? YES NO

12. Do you think that you worry about your health more than most people? YES NO

13. Do you think there is something seriously wrong with your body? YES NO

14. Are you afraid of illness? YES NO

Note. Score 1 point for every YES circled, except for question 9 where 1 point is scored for circling NO. Reprinted with kind permission from Professor Issy Pilowsky, Department of Psychiatry, University of Adelaide, South Australia 5001, Australia.

Worksheet 1. Symptom Interpretation Form

Day and date	Symptom	Initial thoughts	Intensity of anxiety (0–100)	Response	Medical opinion	Scenario
Example	Heart racing and shortness of breath	Believed I was having a heart attack	90	Rushed to emergency room	Nothing wrong. Likely an anxiety attack	False alarm
Example	Headache and sore eyes	Thought it might be a brain tumor but more likely a cold	25	Went to doctor the next day	Sinus infection	Hit (for the cold)
Example	Lumps in right breast	Thought I had breast cancer	99	Visited several doctors and specialists	Harmless fibroids	False alarm

Worksheet 2. Common Stressors

Stress is a fact of life, although people commonly fail to recognize how it affects them. This is because stressors are often minor irritants or hassles. When hassles do occur, people often experience stress-related bodily sensations. This is especially likely when many stressors occur at the same time or in succession. The following are some common stressors. Circle the ones that you experienced in the past week.

Household

Difficulty arranging child care
Too many household chores
Shopping problems
Crowded living space
Difficulties with home maintenance
Misplacing or losing things
Conflicts with partner or children
Divorce or separation
Car trouble

Social

Too few friends
Feeling isolated
Friends or relatives living too far away
Arguments with friends
Dating problems
Unwanted social obligations

Neighborhood and environment

Weather (for example, too hot, too cold, too humid)
Things that you are allergic to
Pollution
Crime
Traffic
Commuting
Noise
Waiting lines
Neighborhood crowding
Troublesome neighbors
Inconsiderate smokers
Parking problems
Problems with other drivers
Discrimination or harassment
Disturbing news stories

Work

Difficult duties
Inadequate training
Lack of a clear job description
Lack of appreciation
No avenue to voice concerns
Insufficient resources
Boring job
Doing job below level of competence
Concerns about shift work
Insufficient backup
Long work hours
A lot of responsibility with little or no authority
Unrealistic deadlines or expectations
Conflict with coworkers
Incompetent colleagues
Hassles from boss
Problems with supervisees
Staff shortages
Difficult clients
Computer problems (hardware or software)
Difficulty keeping up with technological developments
Poor promotional prospects
Unpleasant working conditions (for example, noisy, dirty, no privacy, cramped)
Too much travel (for example, to meetings)
Lack of work boundaries (that is, being contacted after hours by e-mail, phone, or pager)
Corporate downsizing, restructuring, or job relocation
Workplace violence
Lack of job security
Unemployment

(cont.)

Source: From S. Taylor and G. J. G. Asmundson (2004). *Treating health anxiety: A cognitive-behavioral approach*. New York: Guilford Press. Reprinted by permission in *It's Not All in Your Head* by Gordon J. G. Asmundson and Steven Taylor. Copyright 2005 by The Guilford Press. Permission to photocopy this worksheet is granted to purchasers of this book for personal use only (see copyright page for details).

School or university

Conflicts with roommates
Conflicts with other students or instructors
Academic deadlines
Difficult or boring courses
Too much schoolwork
Concerns about career path
Financial problems (for example, problems
   with student loans)
Budgeting problems

Finances

Debts
Credit problems
Lack of money to pay bills
Insufficient money for recreational activities
   (for example, movies)
Problems with taxes
Retirement concerns
Auto payments

Time pressures

Too much to do
Too little to do
Too many interruptions
Insufficient time for recreation
Too many meetings
Too many responsibilities

Health

Physical illness
Physical disability
Concerns with medical treatment
Treatment side effects
Concerns about physical appearance
Overweight
Underweight
Sexual problems

Inner concerns

Inability to express oneself
Conflicts about life choices (for example,
   career, choice of dating partner)
Too much time on one's hands
Concerns about the meaning of life
Too little sleep

Legal

Parking tickets
Speeding fines
Other legal problems

_____

_____

_____

_____

_____

_____

_____

Worksheet 3. Common Stress-Related Bodily Reactions

Stressors, big and small, can produce bodily reactions. Sometimes these reactions happen while you are experiencing a stressful event, and sometimes they occur later on. The following is a list of some of the common stress-related bodily reactions. Not all of these sensations occur together; people typically experience one or two (or sometimes more) of these sensations during times of stress. Circle the ones that you have experienced in the past week. For each bodily sensation you circled, rate how much it bothered you over the past week by placing a number from 1 (*not very bothersome*) to 10 (*extremely bothersome*) on the line beside the sensation.

_____ Muscle spasms	_____ Stomach cramps
_____ Chest pain	_____ Nausea
_____ Feeling restless or fidgety	_____ Indigestion
_____ Fatigue	_____ Stomach churning
_____ Headache	_____ Diarrhea
_____ Neck pain	_____ Frequent need to urinate
_____ Chest tightness	_____ Difficulty swallowing
_____ Leg cramps	_____ Weight gain
_____ Backache	_____ Weight loss
_____ Aches and pains	_____ Heart thumping
_____ Trembling	_____ Heart racing
_____ Difficulty taking a deep breath	_____ Heart skipping a beat
_____ Tingling in the feet or hands	_____ Dry mouth
_____ Muscle twitches	_____ Dizziness
_____ Hot flashes	_____ Feeling light-headed
_____ Sweating	_____ Insomnia

Worksheet 4. A 12-Step Approach to Problem Solving

There are solutions to most of life's problems. The chances of effectively solving your problems depend on the approach you take. The following steps increase the chances of solving important problems in your life.

1. **Pick a problem** that you would like to work on. It could be a big, urgent problem that may take some effort to solve, or it might be a little one. Successfully tackling small problems can increase your confidence of solving bigger problems. List your problem as specifically as possible:

   _____

2. **State your goal.** Please be as specific as possible. What is the outcome that you are hoping to attain? For example, if you are an unemployed accountant, your goal might be to find a full-time accounting position.

   _____

   _____

   _____

3. **Is your goal realistic?** If not, list another, more attainable goal.

   _____

4. **What are your resources for attaining your goal?** This would include material resources (for example, money, transportation) and social resources (for example, people who could help you or offer support).

   _____

   _____

   _____

5. **Brainstorm!** List all the possible ways of attaining your goal that you can think of. List these possibilities regardless of whether they're plausible or not. Use an extra sheet if necessary.

   _____

   _____

   _____

6. **Refine your solutions.** Look through your list of solutions and see if you can think of ways of improving your solutions. If you think of extra solutions while doing this, then write them down as well.

   _____

   _____

   _____

(cont.)

Source: From S. Taylor and G. J. G. Asmundson (2004). *Treating health anxiety: A cognitive-behavioral approach*. New York: Guilford Press. Reprinted by permission in *It's Not All in Your Head* by Gordon J. G. Asmundson and Steven Taylor. Copyright 2005 by The Guilford Press. Permission to photocopy this worksheet is granted to purchasers of this book for personal use only (see copyright page for details).

7. **Evaluate.** List the pros and cons of each solution. Which one looks the best?

_____

_____

_____

_____

8. **Baby steps.** Can you break your goal up into subgoals? For example, if your goal was to find a dating partner, your subgoals might be the following: (a) Put yourself in situations in which you will meet people whom you might like to date (for example, join a sporting club or enroll in a course at a community center). (b) Get to know people. Make friends. Even if you don't find a dating partner, at least you'll have friends. (c) If you find someone attractive, arrange to have coffee with him or her . . . and so on.

_____

_____

_____

_____

9. **Identify obstacles.** What are the things that might get in the way of solving your problems? These might be behavioral obstacles (for example, lack of job skills) or thinking obstacles (for example, negative thoughts such as "Nobody would ever hire me."). List your obstacles here.

_____

_____

_____

_____

10. **Overcome your roadblocks.** List ways of overcoming the obstacles. This might involve improving your skills or challenging your negative thoughts.

_____

_____

_____

_____

11. **Make a commitment** to solving your problems. Plan to do something each day.

12. **Track your progress** toward achieving your goals. Are you making steady progress? If so, good. If not, then identify the roadblocks and try to come up with solutions. Sometimes it helps to reward yourself for your efforts in overcoming problems, especially big problems. Treat yourself to something nice.

Worksheet 5.
Identifying Overgeneralizations and Emotional Reasoning

Symptom/situation	Overgeneralization
Headache	This headache means I must have a brain tumor.
Touching doorknobs	If I touch doorknobs, I'll catch some nasty infectious disease.

Your feelings	Emotional reasoning
Anxious and on edge	I must be sick, otherwise I wouldn't feel so anxious.

Worksheet 6.
Details of a Recent Health Anxiety Episode

One of My Recent Episodes of Health Anxiety

Worksheet 7. Health Anxiety Thoughts and Behaviors Monitoring Form

Day and date	Health anxiety trigger (for example, an event or bodily sensation)	Specific thoughts (and strength of belief from 0 to 100 percent)	Intensity of anxiety (0–100)	What you did to deal with your anxiety.
Tuesday at 6:35 p.m.	Saw a TV program on breast cancer.	Worried that small lumps in my breasts were cancerous. (Believed it 100 percent.)	95	Checked my body for more lumps. Checked so much that my breasts were tender and sore.

Source: From S. Taylor and G. J. G. Asmundson (2004). *Treating health anxiety: A cognitive-behavioral approach.* New York: Guilford Press. Reprinted by permission in *It's Not All in Your Head* by Gordon J. G. Asmundson and Steven Taylor. Copyright 2005 by The Guilford Press. Permission to photocopy this worksheet is granted to purchasers of this book for personal use only (see copyright page for details).

Worksheet 8. Collecting Evidence for and against Specific Thoughts about Health

	Evidence for the specific thought	Evidence against the specific thought
Frightening thought *Example: "The spot on my hand is skin cancer."*		
Alternative explanation *Example: "The spot on my hand is simply a freckle."*		

Worksheet 9. Acceptable Uncertainties in My Life

Uncertainties that the authors of this book are prepared to accept:

- *Commuting to work, even though there's a small chance we could be killed in a car accident.*
- *Eating chicken wings, even though there's a tiny chance we could choke to death on a bone.*
- *Smoking the occasional cigar, even though nobody can guarantee that it's safe.*
- *Flying on a plane, even though it could conceivably crash.*
- *Working the occasional day at home, even though nobody can guarantee that a satellite or piece of space junk won't fall from the sky and crash through one of our roofs.*
- *Shopping in the mall, even though there's no guarantee that a crazed gunman won't kill us all.*
- *Talking on a cell phone, even though no one can give a 110 percent assurance that the electromagnetic waves from the phones are safe.*

Which uncertainties are you prepared to accept? Write them here:

Worksheet 10. Putting You in the Doctor's Shoes

You as the patient	You as the doctor, responding to the patient
Write your real-life health anxieties in this column—that is, the things about your health that you really worry about these days.	Now, put on your white coat and write down the most likely cause of the patient's concerns. Remember, your mission is to make sure that your patient doesn't become needlessly worried about his or her health.
I ate beef last week. Now I'm worried about getting the human version of mad cow disease.	I ate beef, too. So did millions of people. The chances of getting sick are over a million to one. Your time on this earth is too precious for you to be worrying about rare diseases. I suggest that you spend your time on the things that give you a sense of happiness or pride; for example, pursuing fun hobbies, working on a career, or spending quality time with your friends or family.
Lately I've been feeling tired all the time. I'm frightened that I might have AIDS.	Remember that you've already had an HIV test and a number of other medical tests. The most likely causes of fatigue are stress, sleep difficulties, lack of physical fitness, boredom, and too much coffee. When you worry about feeling tired, then you might say this to yourself: "I'm very good at thinking of bad causes of tiredness, but maybe I need to think about all the harmless things that could be making me feel this way. I'll wait and see how I feel in a week or so, before consulting a doctor."
You as the patient:	You as the doctor:
You as the patient:	You as the doctor:
You as the patient:	You as the doctor:

Worksheet 11.
My Checking and Reassurance-Seeking Behaviors

Type	What I do
Bodily checking	
Searching for information	
Reassurance seeking	

Worksheet 12.
Collecting Evidence of Advantages and Disadvantages
of My Checking and Reassurance Seeking Behaviors

	Advantages	Disadvantages
Behavior *Example: "I check the mole on my arm throughout the day, poking and picking at it to see if it's changed color or grown."*		
Alternative behavior *Example: "I could stop checking the mole" or "I could start checking more often, say every two hours for the next four days."*		

Worksheet 13. Monitoring Form for Behavioral Exercises.

Day and date	Exercise	Peak anxiety (0–100)	What did you learn from the exercise?
Example 1	Spent 5 min feeling the lymph glands on neck, to see if they were swollen	50	Repeated checking and squeezing makes my glands feel sore and swollen. Repeated checking creates problems— it makes me think my glands are swollen.
Example 2	Jogged around the block	70	I was worried that my body couldn't take the exertion. But I survived! Maybe I'm not as frail as I thought.
Example 3	Walked past a funeral home	65	Nothing bad happened. I can't get sick by being near dead bodies.

Source: From S. Taylor and G. J. G. Asmundson (2004). *Treating health anxiety: A cognitive-behavioral approach.* New York: Guilford Press. Reprinted by permission in *It's Not All in Your Head* by Gordon J. G. Asmundson and Steven Taylor. Copyright 2005 by The Guilford Press. Permission to photocopy this worksheet is granted to purchasers of this book for personal use only (see copyright page for details).

Worksheet 14.
Things Related to Situations I'm Afraid of

Situation: _____

Worksheet 15. *When to Visit the Doctor*

Instructions: Answer the questions below. Make an appointment with your doctor to discuss the things you've listed. Have him or her assist you in completing the list of confirmed medical illnesses that you should keep an eye on. Working together, come up with a list of times when you should visit the doctor.

Write down all anxiety-related bodily sensations or changes you have. Looking back at worksheets from other chapters may help.

Write down any bodily sensations or symptoms you have that you haven't been able to explain.

What confirmed medical illness do you have? Are regular check-ups for any of these necessary? List check-up frequency for each.

(cont.)

List all legitimate reasons for seeing your doctor here.

I'll visit my family doctor at these times:

- When I have a scheduled annual medical examination.

- When I need inoculations.

- If I need to renew a prescription.

- When I experience bodily sensations that are clearly not normal and don't seem to be part of the stress reaction (for example, blood in my urine, loss of continence, inability to speak).

- _____

- _____

- _____

- _____

- _____

- _____

- _____

- _____

- _____

- _____

- _____

Worksheet 16. *Activities for Enhancing Your Quality of Life*

Instructions: Enjoyable activities are essential to your quality of life. But sometimes people neglect these activities when preoccupied or worried about their health. Look through the following checklist of activities. Did you do any of them in the past week? If so, did you enjoy it? Are there any activities that you haven't done but would like to do? This list might help you think about ways of improving your quality of life.

Activities unrelated to health worries	Indicate (√) which activities you did in the past week.	Were these activities enjoyable? (yes/no)	Indicate (√) which activities you didn't do but would like to do.
Creative activities			
Doing artwork or crafts	_____	_____	_____
Knitting, needlework, sewing	_____	_____	_____
Taking a course in something creative (for example, cooking, photography).	_____	_____	_____
Decorating or redecorating your house or apartment	_____	_____	_____
Woodwork, carpentry, or furniture restoration . . .	_____	_____	_____
Repairing things	_____	_____	_____
Mechanical hobbies (for example, fixing gadgets) .	_____	_____	_____
Photography	_____	_____	_____
Creative writing or doing a journal.	_____	_____	_____
Musical hobbies (for example, singing, dancing, playing an instrument)	_____	_____	_____
Games and entertainment			
Watching TV, videos, or DVDs.	_____	_____	_____
Playing video games	_____	_____	_____
Listening to music or radio programs	_____	_____	_____
Going to the movies.	_____	_____	_____
Going to a play, concert, opera, or ballet	_____	_____	_____
Going to a museum, art gallery, or exhibition . . .	_____	_____	_____
Going to a sporting event	_____	_____	_____
Educational activities that *do not* have to do with gathering information about health and disease			
Reading books, magazines, or newspapers	_____	_____	_____
Going to a lecture on a topic that interests you . .	_____	_____	_____
Learning a foreign language	_____	_____	_____
Surfing the Internet	_____	_____	_____
Learning about computers (for example, learning to make a Web page)	_____	_____	_____
Going to the library	_____	_____	_____

(*cont.*)

Source: From S. Taylor and G. J. G. Asmundson (2004). *Treating health anxiety: A cognitive-behavioral approach*. New York: Guilford Press. Reprinted by permission in *It's Not All in Your Head* by Gordon J. G. Asmundson and Steven Taylor. Copyright 2005 by The Guilford Press. Permission to photocopy this worksheet is granted to purchasers of this book for personal use only (see copyright page for details).

	Did do:	Enjoyable?	Want to do:
Physical activities			
Playing tennis, squash, or racquetball	_____	_____	_____
Playing golf	_____	_____	_____
Ten-pin bowling.	_____	_____	_____
Water activities (for example, swimming, sailing, canoeing)	_____	_____	_____
Walking or hiking	_____	_____	_____
Jogging, aerobics classes, or working out at a fitness center	_____	_____	_____
Snow sports (skiing, skating, snowboarding)	_____	_____	_____
Bike riding	_____	_____	_____
Horseback riding	_____	_____	_____
Playing team sports (for example, volleyball, hockey, basketball)	_____	_____	_____
Fishing or hunting.	_____	_____	_____
Playing snooker or pool	_____	_____	_____
Social and community activities that *do not* involve discussing health and disease			
Writing, telephoning, or e-mailing friends.	_____	_____	_____
Visiting a friend or inviting a friend to your place	_____	_____	_____
Going out to lunch or dinner with a friend	_____	_____	_____
Giving a party or going to a party	_____	_____	_____
Going on a date	_____	_____	_____
Joining a club (for example, a book club or social club) . .	_____	_____	_____
Going to a bar or restaurant	_____	_____	_____
Involvement in community or political activities	_____	_____	_____
Involvement in religious or church activities.	_____	_____	_____
Other			
Sitting in the sun	_____	_____	_____
Going for a scenic drive	_____	_____	_____
Gardening, caring for houseplants, or arranging flowers . .	_____	_____	_____
Visiting fun or interesting places (for example, park, beach, zoo)	_____	_____	_____
Caring for or being with pets	_____	_____	_____
Planning or going on a vacation.	_____	_____	_____
Going to a sauna	_____	_____	_____
Soaking in the bathtub	_____	_____	_____
Doing yoga or meditation.	_____	_____	_____
Buying yourself something special.	_____	_____	_____
Hobbies (for example, stamp collecting, model building, flying a kite)	_____	_____	_____
List your favorite activities here, if they are not listed above:			
_____	_____	_____	_____
_____	_____	_____	_____
_____	_____	_____	_____
_____	_____	_____	_____

Worksheet 17. Activity Enjoyment Rating Form

Instructions: List each activity you do for enjoyment over the next few weeks. Rate the enjoyment the activity brings you using a scale with 0 = no enjoyment and 4 = a lot of enjoyment.

Day and date	Activity	Enjoyment rating
Example	Went to a movie	3
Example	Took my kids to play in the park	4

Index

About the Authors

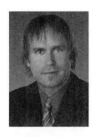

Gordon J. G. Asmundson, PhD, is Professor and Canadian Institutes of Health Research Investigator in Psychology and Kinesiology and Health Studies at the University of Regina, Canada, and Adjunct Professor of Psychiatry at the University of Saskatchewan. He is currently North American Editor of *Cognitive Behaviour Therapy,* Behavioral Medicine Section Editor for *Cognitive and Behavioral Practice,* PTSD Section Coeditor for *Psychological Injury and Law,* and serves on the editorial boards for the *Journal of Anxiety Disorders,* the *Journal of Behavior Therapy and Experimental Psychiatry,* the *Clinical Journal of Pain,* and several other journals. He has published over 220 journal articles and book chapters, as well as six books, including *Clinical Research in Mental Health* (with G. Ron Norton and Murray B. Stein; 2001, Thousand Oaks, CA: Sage), the edited volume *Health Anxiety* (with Steven Taylor and Brian J. Cox; 2001, New York: Wiley), and the coauthored volume *Treating Health Anxiety: A Cognitive-Behavioral Approach* (with Steven Taylor; 2004, New York: Guilford Press). He served as a member of the *Diagnostic and Statistical Manual of Mental Disorders, Fourth Edition, Text Revision* Work Group for the Anxiety Disorders. Dr. Asmundson's research contributions have been recognized by early career awards from the Anxiety Disorders Association of America, the Canadian chapter of the International Association for the Study of Pain, and the Canadian Psychological Association. Most recently, he was elected to status of Fellow in the Royal Society of Canada in recognition of his pioneering work on the overlap between the anxiety disorders and chronic pain. He is actively involved in clinical research and clinical research supervision and has interests in assessment and basic mechanisms of the anxiety disorders, health anxiety, acute and chronic pain, and the association of these with disability and behavior change.

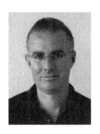

Steven Taylor, PhD, ABPP, is a clinical psychologist and Professor in the Department of Psychiatry at the University of British Columbia, Canada. He received his graduate training at the University of Melbourne, Australia, and the University of British Columbia. Dr. Taylor is board certified in cognitive and behavioral psychology by the American Board of Professional Psychology. For 10 years he was Associate Editor of *Behaviour Research and Therapy* and is now Editor-in-Chief of the *Journal of Cognitive Psychotherapy.* He serves on the editorial boards of several journals, including the *Journal of Consulting and Clinical Psychology* and the *Journal of Abnormal Psychology.* Dr. Taylor has published over 200 journal articles and book chapters. He has also published over 15 books on anxiety disorders and related topics. He served as a consultant on the *Diagnostic and Statistical Manual of Mental Disorders, Fourth Edition, Text Revision*. Dr. Taylor has received career awards from the Canadian Psychological Association, the British Columbia Psychological Association, the Association for Advancement of Behavior Therapy, and the Anxiety Disorders Association of America. He is a Fellow of several scholarly organizations, including the Canadian Psychological Association, the American Psychological Association, the Association for Psychological Science, and the Academy of Cognitive Therapy. Dr. Taylor's research interests include cognitive-behavioral treatments and mechanisms of anxiety disorders and related conditions, as well as the behavioral genetics of these disorders. His research has been funded by grants from the Canadian Institutes of Health Research.